COOKING FOR PCOS WELLNESS

Nurturing Your Body with Satisfying and Nourishing Recipes

Lenore G. Stevens

Copyright © 2023 by Lenore G. Stevens

TABLE OF CONTENT

INTRODUCTION

In a bustling city, Olivia, a young woman on a quest for renewed health and balance, stumbled upon a remarkable book that would transform her life. "Cooking for PCOS Wellness: Nurturing Your Body with Satisfying and Nourishing Recipes" beckoned to her, promising a path towards managing her Polycystic Ovary Syndrome (PCOS) and embracing a nourishing lifestyle.

As Olivia delved into the pages of this captivating cookbook, she discovered a world of vibrant flavors, nutrient-rich ingredients, and culinary wisdom tailored specifically for PCOS individuals. The book offered more than just recipes; it was a guide to reclaiming control over her body and fostering overall well-being.

From energizing breakfasts to wholesome lunches, satisfying dinners, and delightful snacks, each recipe was thoughtfully crafted to support hormone balance, provide essential nutrients, and tantalize her taste buds. Olivia found solace in the pages, knowing that she could now nourish her body with delicious and PCOS-friendly meals.

The benefits of this newfound approach to cooking and eating soon became evident. Olivia experienced increased energy levels, improved mood, and a newfound sense of empowerment. She discovered the power of mindful eating, savoring each bite and forging a deeper connection with her body's needs.

Not only did the book offer tantalizing recipes, but it also provided valuable insights into the role of nutrition in managing PCOS symptoms. Olivia learned about essential nutrients and the importance of balanced meal planning. Armed with this knowledge, she confidently navigated the grocery store, stocking her pantry with PCOS-friendly ingredients and making informed choices.

As Olivia embarked on her PCOS wellness journey, she realized that this cookbook was more than just a collection of recipes; it was a trusted companion, guiding her towards a healthier, more fulfilling life. Cooking became a joyful act of self-care, a way to honor her body and nourish her soul.

With each meal she prepared from the book, Olivia celebrated her journey towards PCOS wellness. The book became her secret weapon, empowering her to reclaim control over her health and embrace a vibrant, fulfilling life.

Today, Olivia is a shining example of the transformative power of cooking for PCOS wellness. She shares her story with others, spreading the word about the benefits of this remarkable book and inspiring individuals with PCOS to embark on their own culinary journeys towards healing and self-discovery.

"Cooking for PCOS Wellness: Nurturing Your Body with Satisfying and Nourishing Recipes" continues to touch the lives of countless individuals, guiding them towards renewed health, vitality, and a deep appreciation for the nourishment that comes from within.

Step into this culinary adventure, embrace the flavors, and unlock the incredible benefits of cooking for PCOS wellness. Your journey awaits.

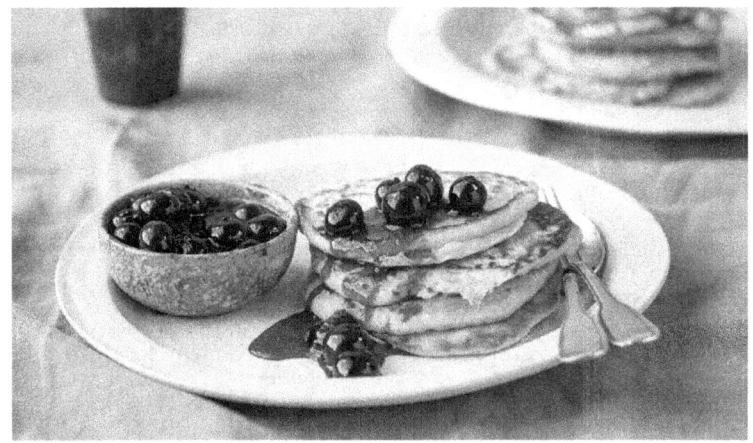

CHAPTER 1

Polycystic Ovary Syndrome (PCOS) is a complicated hormonal condition that affects millions of people, primarily women of reproductive age. Living with PCOS may bring unique issues, including irregular menstrual periods, hormone abnormalities, weight swings, and difficulty with conception.

However, by having a greater awareness of PCOS and the importance of diet in controlling its symptoms, persons with PCOS may empower themselves to take charge of their health and well-being.

In this book, we will investigate the complicated link between PCOS and nutrition. We will go into what PCOS is, how it affects the body, and why taking a mindful approach to eating is vital for controlling its symptoms. By acquiring insights into the influence of diet on PCOS, we may make educated decisions regarding the foods we eat, leveraging their potential to ease symptoms and enhance overall wellbeing.

PCOS alters the delicate balance of hormones in the body, resulting to a variety of physical and emotional symptoms. Irregular menstrual periods, increased androgen production, insulin resistance, and weight gain are just some of the issues that patients with PCOS may experience. While there is no treatment for PCOS, adopting a healthy lifestyle that includes a well-balanced diet may greatly improve symptoms and boost quality of life.

Nutrition plays a vital role in controlling PCOS symptoms by addressing underlying hormonal imbalances, supporting weight management, lowering inflammation, and increasing insulin sensitivity. Through focused dietary choices, persons with PCOS may control their hormone levels, stabilize blood sugar levels, manage their weight, and lower the risk of long-term consequences associated with the disorder.

We will review key foods that are especially useful for persons with PCOS. We will examine the role of fiber, omega-3 fatty acids, antioxidants, chromium, and vitamin D in controlling PCOS symptoms and boosting general well-being. Additionally, we will give practical direction on developing a balanced PCOS-friendly diet, stressing the integration of complex carbs, lean proteins, healthy fats, fruits, and vegetables.

It is crucial to remember that every person with PCOS is unique, and what works for one individual may not work for another. The road to understanding PCOS and diet is a personal one that involves patience, self-awareness, and experimentation. By listening to your body, recording how various meals make you feel, and getting expert help when required, you can adapt your diet to meet your individual requirements and objectives.

Through this detailed study of PCOS and nutrition, we welcome you to go on a transformational journey of knowledge, self-discovery, and empowerment.

By embracing the power of nutrition, you can take charge of your health, lessen PCOS symptoms, and pave the road for a bright and full life.

What is PCOS and how does it affect your body?

Polycystic Ovary Syndrome (PCOS) is a complicated hormonal condition that affects many people, mainly women of reproductive age.

It is characterized by a variety of symptoms, including irregular menstrual periods, hormonal abnormalities, cysts on the ovaries, and insulin resistance. PCOS may have a dramatic influence on physical and mental well-being, frequently presenting issues in different parts of life, including fertility, weight management, and general health.

PCOS alters the natural hormonal balance in the body, resulting to an overproduction of androgens, generally known as male hormones. This hormonal imbalance may result in irregular or nonexistent menstrual cycles, as well as the formation of tiny cysts on the ovaries.

Additionally, PCOS commonly corresponds with insulin resistance, a disease in which the body's cells become less receptive to the hormone insulin, leading to high blood sugar levels.

The importance of diet in controlling PCOS symptoms:

While PCOS is a lifelong diagnosis, the good news is that adopting a healthy lifestyle, including a well-balanced diet, may considerably reduce symptoms and improve overall well-being.

Nutrition plays a significant role in controlling PCOS symptoms by helping to balance hormone levels, improve weight management, decrease inflammation, and increase insulin sensitivity.

One of the primary dietary issues for PCOS persons is keeping stable blood sugar levels. The prevalence of insulin resistance in PCOS may lead to high insulin levels, which can drive androgen production and worsen hormonal imbalances. Therefore, concentrating on a diet that helps manage blood sugar levels might be advantageous.

5 Essential nutrients for PCOS individuals:

Incorporating certain nutrients into your diet might be especially useful in treating PCOS symptoms. Here are some crucial nutrients to consider:

1. Fiber: Consuming an appropriate quantity of dietary fiber is beneficial for those with PCOS. Fiber helps balance blood sugar levels, improves fullness, assists in weight management, and supports good digestion. Good sources of fiber include fruits, vegetables, whole grains, legumes, and seeds.

2. Omega-3 fatty acids: These important fats have been demonstrated to lower inflammation in the body, which might be useful for those with PCOS, since inflammation is commonly present. Foods high in omega-3 fatty acids include fatty fish (such as salmon and sardines), flaxseeds, chia seeds, and walnuts.

3. Antioxidants: Including a range of antioxidant-rich foods in your diet will help prevent oxidative stress and inflammation linked with PCOS.

Colorful fruits and vegetables, such as berries, leafy greens, bell peppers, and tomatoes, are good providers of antioxidants.

4. Chromium: This mineral has a function in controlling blood sugar levels and enhancing insulin sensitivity. Good dietary sources of chromium include broccoli, green beans, whole grains, and almonds.

5. Vitamin D: Many persons with PCOS have been discovered to have low levels of vitamin D. Adequate vitamin D consumption is vital for hormonal balance and general health. Natural sources of vitamin D include sunshine exposure, fatty fish, fortified dairy products, and egg yolks.

Building a balanced PCOS-friendly diet:

When it comes to developing a balanced diet for PCOS, focusing on nutrient-dense whole foods is crucial. Here are 10 recommendations to help you build a PCOS-friendly diet plan:

1. **Prioritize complex carbs:** Choose whole grains, such as quinoa, brown rice, and oats, over processed carbohydrates. Complex carbs give lasting energy and help normalize blood sugar levels.

2. **Include lean proteins:** Opt for lean sources of protein, such as chicken, fish, lentils, and tofu. Protein is vital for hormone production, muscular maintenance, and increasing satiety.

3. **Embrace good fats:** Incorporate sources of healthy fats, such as avocados, nuts, seeds, and olive oil, into your diet. Healthy fats enhance satiety, boost hormone synthesis, and help in nutrition absorption.

4. **Load up on fruits and veggies:** Fill your plate with a colorful variety of fruits and vegetables, since they are high in antioxidants, fiber, and important vitamins and minerals.

5. **Practice portion control:** Pay attention to portion sizes to ensure you're ingesting a suitable quantity of calories for

your specific requirements. Overeating may lead to weight gain, which can worsen PCOS symptoms.

6. Stay hydrated: Drink lots of water throughout the day to promote general hydration and enhance body processes.

7. Minimize processed foods and added sugars: Processed meals, sugary snacks, and drinks may induce blood sugar increases and lead to weight gain. Limiting their intake may assist manage insulin levels and maintain a healthy weight.

8. Be aware of dairy intake: Some persons with PCOS may be sensitive to dairy products. Consider experimenting with alternate alternatives like almond milk, coconut milk, or soy milk and observe how your body reacts.

9. Incorporate PCOS-specific foods: Certain foods have been discovered to be especially useful for those with PCOS. For example, spearmint tea has showed promise in decreasing testosterone levels, whereas cinnamon has been related with increased insulin sensitivity.

10. Consider professional guidance: Consulting with a licensed dietitian or nutritionist who specializes in PCOS may give tailored suggestions and assistance. They can help you build a personalized food plan that matches your unique requirements, tastes, and objectives.

It's crucial to remember that every person with PCOS is unique, and what works for one individual may not work for another. It may take some trial and error to understand which dietary practices and particular foods best support your health and ease your symptoms.

Listening to your body, recording how various meals make you feel, and making modifications appropriately is crucial.

In addition to diet, including regular physical exercise, stress management strategies, and appropriate sleep into your lifestyle will further increase your general well-being and PCOS treatment.

Understanding the delicate link between PCOS and diet allows you to make educated decisions that promote your health and quality of life. By developing a balanced PCOS-friendly diet, you may optimize hormone balance, control weight, increase insulin sensitivity, and decrease inflammation.

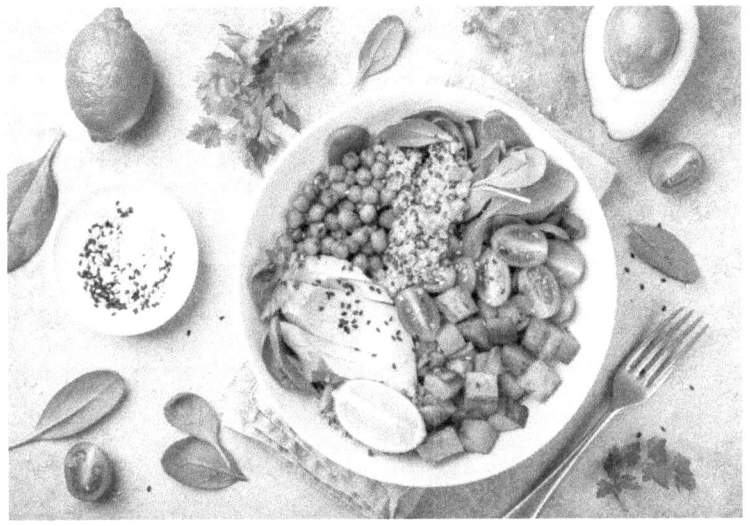

CHAPTER 2

L iving with Polycystic Ovary Syndrome (PCOS) can present unique challenges, particularly when it comes to managing weight, hormonal imbalances, and emotional well-being. In the pursuit of holistic health, incorporating mindful eating practices can be a powerful tool for individuals with PCOS to nourish their bodies, cultivate a positive relationship with food, and enhance overall well-being.

PCOS is a complex hormonal disorder that affects many aspects of a person's health, including metabolism, insulin resistance, and reproductive health. One of the key factors in managing PCOS is adopting a mindful approach to eating, which involves being fully present and attentive to the eating experience.

Mindful eating encourages individuals to pay attention to their body's hunger and fullness cues, to savor and appreciate the flavors and textures of food, and to make conscious choices that align with their health goals.

In this chapter, we will explore the intersection of PCOS and mindful eating, and how it can support individuals in their journey towards optimal wellness. We will delve into the practice of mindfulness and its application to various aspects of eating, including meal planning, emotional eating, portion control, and building a positive relationship with food and the body.

Practicing mindfulness in your eating habits can help you develop a deeper understanding of your body's needs and responses to different foods. By bringing awareness to the present moment, you can make conscious decisions about the quality and quantity of food you consume. Mindful eating also enables you to tune in to your body's signals of hunger and fullness, allowing for a more balanced and intuitive approach to nourishing yourself.

For persons with PCOS, emotional eating may be a typical challenge. Stress, anxiety, and other emotional triggers can lead to a disconnection from physical hunger cues and an overreliance on food for emotional comfort. This chapter will provide strategies to overcome emotional eating challenges, including identifying triggers, developing alternative coping mechanisms, and practicing self-compassion.

By addressing emotional eating patterns, individuals can develop a healthier relationship with food and better manage their PCOS symptoms.

Portion control is another crucial aspect of managing PCOS, as it helps maintain a healthy weight and supports insulin sensitivity. Mindful eating techniques can aid in portion control by promoting awareness of portion sizes, encouraging slower eating, and allowing individuals to truly savor and enjoy their meals. We will explore practical strategies for incorporating portion control mindfully into daily life, making mealtime a balanced and satisfying experience.

Building a positive relationship with food and the body is essential for overall well-being, especially for individuals with PCOS who may experience body image issues or feelings of guilt and shame surrounding food. Mindful eating emphasizes self-acceptance, body positivity, and self-care, promoting a compassionate and non-judgmental attitude towards oneself and one's body.

This book will offer guidance on cultivating body appreciation, practicing self-compassion, and embracing intuitive eating principles.

By integrating mindful eating practices into their lives, individuals with PCOS can harness the power of food as a tool for nourishment, healing, and self-care. Mindful eating empowers individuals to make informed choices, honor their bodies' unique needs, and cultivate a positive relationship with food. It is a journey of self-discovery, self-compassion, and embracing the present moment.

We will explore the concept of mindful eating and provide strategies to overcome emotional eating challenges, practice portion control, and build a positive and nourishing relationship with food.

Practicing Mindfulness in Your Eating Habits:

Mindful eating begins with cultivating awareness and presence during meals. By slowing down and savoring each bite, we can reconnect with the sensory experience of eating. This section will guide you through various techniques to practice mindfulness while eating, such as mindful chewing, engaging your senses, and creating mindful meal rituals.

By paying attention to the textures, flavors, and aromas of your food, you can enhance your eating experience and develop a deeper appreciation for the nourishment it provides.

Overcoming Emotional Eating Challenges:

Emotional eating is a common struggle for many individuals, and it can be particularly challenging for those with PCOS. Stress, anxiety, boredom, or other negative emotions can trigger the urge to seek comfort in food, leading to overeating and potential weight gain.

This section will explore strategies to overcome emotional eating challenges by identifying emotional triggers, developing alternative coping mechanisms, and practicing self-compassion.

By addressing the underlying emotional issues, you can break free from the cycle of emotional eating and develop a healthier relationship with food.

Strategies for Mindful Meal Planning and Portion Control:

Mindful meal planning and portion control are crucial for managing PCOS and supporting a healthy lifestyle. This section will provide practical strategies for incorporating mindfulness into your meal planning process. You will learn how to engage in mindful grocery shopping, choose nutrient-dense foods, and create balanced meals that meet your nutritional needs.

We will also explore portion control techniques, such as using visual cues, practicing mindful eating pauses, and listening to your body's hunger and fullness signals. By practicing portion control mindfully, you can maintain a healthy weight and optimize your PCOS management.

Building a Healthy Relationship with Food and Your Body: Developing a healthy relationship with food and your body is essential for long-term well-being. This section will delve into the importance of self-acceptance, body positivity, and self-care in fostering a positive body image.

You will learn strategies to cultivate body appreciation, practice self-compassion, and embrace intuitive eating principles. By shifting your mindset and adopting a holistic approach to wellness, you can develop a harmonious relationship with food and your body, free from guilt and judgment.

By incorporating mindful eating practices into your daily life, you can transform your relationship with food, enhance your overall well-being, and better manage your PCOS symptoms. Mindful eating allows you to savor the flavors, appreciate the nourishment, and make conscious choices that align with your health goals.

It empowers you to listen to your body's cues, honor your hunger and fullness, and make mindful decisions about what, when, and how you eat.

As you embark on your mindful eating journey, remember that it is a process of self-discovery and self-care. Be gentle with yourself and exercise self-compassion along the process.

Each meal is an opportunity to deepen your connection with your body, nourish yourself, and cultivate a deeper sense of self-awareness. By practicing mindfulness, overcoming emotional eating challenges, mastering portion control, and building a healthy relationship with food and your body, you can create a sustainable and empowering lifestyle that supports your PCOS wellness goals.

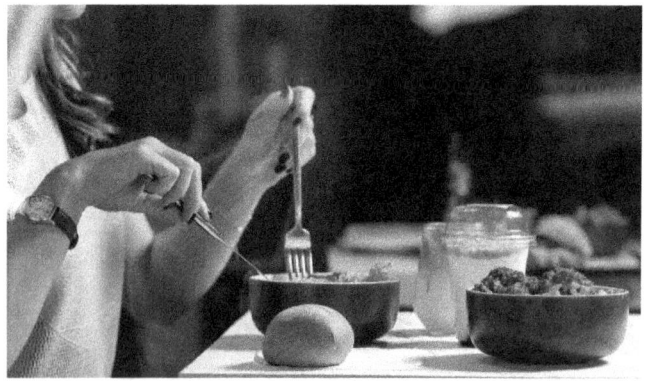

CHAPTER 3

BREAKFAST DELIGHTS

Breakfast is often considered the most important meal of the day, and for individuals with PCOS, it holds even greater significance. A well-balanced and nourishing breakfast can provide a range of benefits, from regulating blood sugar levels to supporting hormone balance and providing sustained energy throughout the day.

In this chapter, we will embark on a culinary journey through a selection of delectable breakfast delights specifically designed with PCOS individuals in mind.

Starting your day with a wholesome and PCOS-friendly breakfast is essential for managing symptoms and promoting overall well-being. The recipes in this chapter are crafted to not only tantalize your taste buds but also deliver a powerful dose of essential nutrients to fuel your body and mind. From energizing smoothie bowls to fluffy gluten-free pancakes, vegetable-packed frittatas, and creamy chia pudding, these breakfast options will nourish your body and set the stage for a vibrant day ahead.

The chapter begins with an exploration of energizing morning smoothie bowls. These bowls are packed with nutrient-rich ingredients like leafy greens, fruits, and plant-based proteins. With their vibrant colors and refreshing flavors, smoothie bowls offer a delightful way to kickstart your day and ensure you get a wide variety of essential nutrients to support your overall well-being.

Next, we delve into the realm of fluffy gluten-free pancakes. Made with alternative flours such as almond or oat flour, these pancakes are not only delicious but also lower in carbohydrates and higher in fiber compared to traditional pancakes.

Topped with a homemade berry compote bursting with antioxidants, these pancakes provide a guilt-free indulgence that won't spike your blood sugar levels.

For those who prefer a savory breakfast, our vegetable-packed frittata recipe will surely please your taste buds. Packed with colorful vegetables, protein-rich eggs, and fragrant herbs, this frittata offers a balanced and satisfying option to fuel your morning. With each bite, you'll be nourishing your body with essential vitamins, minerals, and fiber.

Finally, we explore the convenience of overnight chia pudding. By simply combining chia seeds with milk and a natural sweetener, and allowing it to sit overnight, you can wake up to a creamy and nutritious breakfast option. Topped with an assortment of fresh fruits, this chia pudding provides a boost of omega-3 fatty acids, antioxidants, and fiber to support your PCOS wellness journey.

These breakfast delights are more than just recipes. They represent an invitation to prioritize your health and well-being from the moment you wake up. By incorporating these PCOS-friendly breakfast options into your daily routine, you can nourish your body, support hormone balance, and set the stage for a day filled with vitality and joy.

Breakfast is often hailed as the most important meal of the day, and for individuals with PCOS, it holds even greater significance. Starting your day with a nourishing and balanced breakfast can help regulate blood sugar levels, support hormone balance, and provide sustained energy throughout the day.

We will explore a delightful array of PCOS-friendly breakfast recipes that are not only delicious but also packed with essential nutrients to kickstart your mornings.

Energizing Morning Smoothie Bowl

Smoothie bowls have gained popularity in recent years for their refreshing flavors and vibrant colors. These bowls offer a fantastic opportunity to pack in a wide variety of nutrients from fruits, vegetables, and other nourishing ingredients.

To create an energizing morning smoothie bowl, begin with a base of leafy greens such as spinach or kale, which are rich in fiber, vitamins, and minerals. Add a selection of fruits like berries, bananas, or mangoes, which provide natural sweetness and antioxidants.

To boost the protein content, include a scoop of plant-based protein powder or Greek yogurt. For creaminess, opt for almond milk or coconut milk. Blend the ingredients until smooth and pour the mixture into a bowl.

Top your smoothie bowl with a variety of toppings like sliced fruits, nuts, seeds, and a drizzle of honey or maple syrup for added flavor. This breakfast bowl not only provides a refreshing start to your day but also delivers a range of nutrients to support your overall well-being.

Fluffy Gluten-Free Pancakes with Berry Compote

Pancakes are a classic breakfast option loved by many, and with a few modifications, they can be made PCOS-friendly and gluten-free.

Traditional pancakes are typically made with refined wheat flour, which can cause blood sugar spikes. By using alternative flours such as almond flour or oat flour, you can create fluffy and gluten-free pancakes that are higher in fiber and have a lower glycemic index.

To add natural sweetness and additional nutrients, incorporate mashed bananas or sweet potatoes into the batter. These ingredients provide a dose of vitamins, minerals, and fiber. Once the pancakes are cooked to perfection, serve them with a homemade berry compote. Simply simmer fresh or frozen berries with a squeeze of lemon juice and a touch of natural sweetener like stevia or honey.

The resulting compote is bursting with antioxidants and adds a delightful burst of flavor to your stack of pancakes. This PCOS-friendly breakfast option allows you to indulge in a comforting meal without compromising your health goals.

Vegetable-Packed Frittata with Herbs and Feta

If you prefer a savory breakfast, a vegetable-packed frittata is an excellent choice. This protein-rich dish combines the goodness of eggs with an assortment of colorful vegetables. It not only provides essential nutrients but also keeps you feeling satisfied throughout the morning.

To create a vegetable-packed frittata, start by whisking eggs or egg whites together in a bowl. Chop an array of vegetables such as bell peppers, spinach, zucchini, cherry tomatoes, or any other vegetables you enjoy. Sauté the vegetables in a skillet until they are tender and then pour the beaten eggs over them.

Sprinkle fragrant herbs like basil or thyme and crumble in some feta cheese for added flavor. Transfer the skillet to the oven and bake until the frittata is golden and set.

The end result is a delightful and nutrient-dense breakfast option that combines protein, vitamins, and minerals in a single dish.

Overnight Chia Pudding with Fresh Fruits

For those busy mornings when you need a quick and convenient breakfast option, overnight chia pudding is a perfect choice. Chia seeds are a powerhouse of nutrition, rich in fiber, omega-3 fatty acids, and antioxidants.

To prepare overnight chia pudding, simply combine chia seeds with your choice of milk, such as almond milk or coconut milk.

Sweeten the mixture with a natural sweetener like honey or stevia. Stir well to ensure that the chia seeds are evenly distributed.

Let the mixture sit in the refrigerator overnight, allowing the chia seeds to absorb the liquid and create a thick and creamy pudding-like texture. In the morning, give the pudding a good stir and top it with an assortment of fresh fruits, such as sliced strawberries, blueberries, or kiwi.

The chia seeds provide a satisfying and filling breakfast option, while the fresh fruits add a burst of vitamins, minerals, and natural sweetness.

This make-ahead breakfast allows you to have a nutritious start to your day without sacrificing precious time in the morning.

By incorporating these breakfast delights into your PCOS-friendly meal plan, you can ensure that you nourish your body with essential nutrients, support hormone balance, and set the tone for a productive and energized day.

Experiment with different flavors, textures, and combinations to find the breakfast options that resonate with your taste buds and provide optimal nourishment for your unique needs.

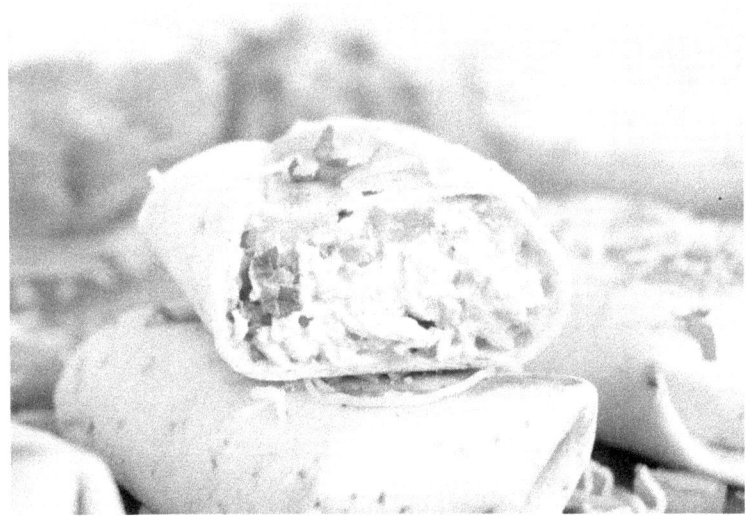

CHAPTER 4

L unchtime is a crucial opportunity to refuel our bodies and provide them with the nourishment they need to power through the day. For individuals with PCOS, crafting a lunch that supports hormone balance, provides essential nutrients, and keeps energy levels stable is of utmost importance.

In this chapter, we will explore the realm of wholesome lunches—delicious and PCOS-friendly meals designed to fuel your body with the right combination of ingredients for optimal well-being.

Wholesome lunches offer an array of benefits, including improved satiety, stable blood sugar levels, and a wealth of essential nutrients.

They are carefully curated to strike the perfect balance of proteins, carbohydrates, healthy fats, and a rainbow of vegetables, ensuring that every bite contributes to your overall wellness.

We will journey through a collection of diverse and delectable lunch recipes that cater to different tastes and dietary preferences. From vibrant salads bursting with flavor to hearty soups and satisfying wraps, these recipes are designed to keep you nourished, satisfied, and energized throughout the day.

Each recipe has been thoughtfully crafted to incorporate ingredients known for their positive effects on PCOS symptoms. We have selected foods that help regulate insulin levels, promote hormonal balance, and support a healthy metabolism.

By choosing these wholesome lunch options, you are not only taking care of your PCOS management but also indulging in delicious meals that prioritize your well-being.

Whether you're seeking a light and refreshing salad packed with nutrient-dense ingredients or a warming and comforting soup to soothe your soul, the recipes in this chapter will inspire you to elevate your lunchtime experience.

Embrace the power of wholesome ingredients, flavors, and textures as you embark on a journey to nourish your body and support your PCOS wellness goals.

By dedicating time and attention to preparing and enjoying these nourishing lunches, you are making a conscious choice to prioritize your health and well-being. Let these recipes guide you toward a balanced and fulfilling lunchtime routine that not only supports your PCOS journey but also brings joy to your taste buds.

As we delve into the world of wholesome lunches, get ready to savor every bite, nourish your body from within, and revel in the pleasure of eating delicious food that promotes your overall wellness.

We will explore a variety of delicious and PCOS-friendly lunch recipes that will not only tantalize your taste buds but also provide a powerful combination of nutrients to support your health.

Quinoa and Roasted Vegetable Salad with Lemon-Tahini Dressing:

A quinoa and roasted vegetable salad is a refreshing and nutritious lunch option. Begin by cooking quinoa until it's fluffy and tender. Meanwhile, roast a medley of colorful vegetables such as bell peppers, zucchini, eggplant, and cherry tomatoes in the oven until they are caramelized and slightly charred.

Combine the cooked quinoa and roasted vegetables in a bowl and drizzle a zesty lemon-tahini dressing over them. The dressing, made with tahini, lemon juice, garlic, and a touch of honey, adds a creamy and tangy flavor. This salad provides a perfect balance of protein, fiber, and vitamins, keeping you satisfied and nourished throughout the day.

Lettuce wraps are a light and refreshing lunch option, and the combination of grilled chicken and avocado is both delicious and nutritious.

Start by marinating chicken breast with a flavorful blend of herbs, spices, and a squeeze of lime juice. Grill the chicken until it's cooked through and has a nice charred exterior. While the chicken is grilling, prepare the avocado spread by mashing ripe avocados with lime juice, salt, and pepper.

Take large lettuce leaves and spread a generous amount of the avocado mixture on each leaf. Place slices of grilled chicken on top and add your favorite toppings like diced tomatoes, cucumbers, and red onions.

These lettuce wraps offer a satisfying dose of lean protein, healthy fats, and fresh vegetables, making them an ideal choice for a light and nutritious lunch.

Sweet Potato and Black Bean Chili:

A hearty and flavorful sweet potato and black bean chili is perfect for those colder days when you crave something warm and comforting.

Begin by sautéing onions, garlic, and spices in a large pot until they become fragrant. Add diced sweet potatoes, black beans, crushed tomatoes, vegetable broth, and a selection of spices.

Let the chili simmer on low heat until the sweet potatoes are tender and the flavors have melded together. This chili is packed with fiber, vitamins, and minerals, and the combination of sweet potatoes and black beans provides a good balance of complex carbohydrates and plant-based protein. Serve the chili with a dollop of Greek yogurt or a sprinkle of fresh herbs for added creaminess and flavor.

This wholesome chili will keep you satisfied and provide a nourishing and satisfying lunch.

Tuna salad gets a Mediterranean twist in this refreshing and protein-packed lunch option. In a bowl, combine canned tuna, diced cucumbers, cherry tomatoes, Kalamata olives, red onions, and crumbled feta cheese.

The combination of flavors from the tangy olives, juicy tomatoes, and creamy feta cheese creates a delightful harmony. For the dressing, whisk together Greek yogurt, lemon juice, fresh herbs like dill or parsley, garlic, and a pinch of salt and pepper.

Drizzle the dressing over the tuna salad mixture and gently toss to coat everything. This Mediterranean-style tuna salad offers a balance of protein, healthy fats, and a medley of fresh vegetables, providing a satisfying and flavorful lunch option.

These wholesome lunch recipes not only cater to your nutritional needs but also offer a diverse range of flavors and textures to keep your taste buds satisfied.

By incorporating these PCOS-friendly lunch options into your meal planning, you can support hormone balance, manage symptoms, and promote overall well-being.

Incorporating quinoa into a salad provides a high-quality source of plant-based protein, while the roasted vegetables add a delicious depth of flavor. The lemon-tahini dressing adds a tangy and creamy element that ties the ingredients together perfectly. This salad is not only satisfying but also rich in fiber, vitamins, and minerals.

The combination of grilled chicken and avocado in lettuce wraps offers a balance of lean protein and healthy fats. Lettuce wraps provide a lighter alternative to bread or tortilla wraps, while still providing a satisfying crunch. The addition of fresh vegetables adds a burst of color and nutrients. These wraps are not only delicious but also contribute to a well-rounded and nourishing lunch.

When it comes to comfort food, the sweet potato and black bean chili is a winner. Packed with fiber, antioxidants, and complex carbohydrates, sweet potatoes provide a nutritious base for this hearty chili. The black beans offer a good source of plant-based protein and fiber, promoting a feeling of fullness and supporting digestive health. The combination of spices and aromatics creates a warm and comforting flavor profile, making it a perfect choice for chilly days or when you need a satisfying and nutritious meal.

For a Mediterranean-inspired lunch, the tuna salad with Greek yogurt dressing is a refreshing and protein-rich option. Tuna provides a lean source of protein, while the fresh vegetables and Greek yogurt dressing offer a cooling and tangy contrast.

The flavors of the olives, tomatoes, and feta cheese transport you to the sunny shores of the Mediterranean. This salad not only satisfies your taste buds but also provides essential nutrients to support your overall wellness.

Incorporating these wholesome lunch options into your meal repertoire will not only support your PCOS management but also promote a healthy and balanced lifestyle.

These recipes prioritize nutrient-dense ingredients, balance macronutrients, and offer a delicious way to nourish your body. By making conscious choices and embracing these flavorful and nutritious meals, you can take charge of your health and well-being.

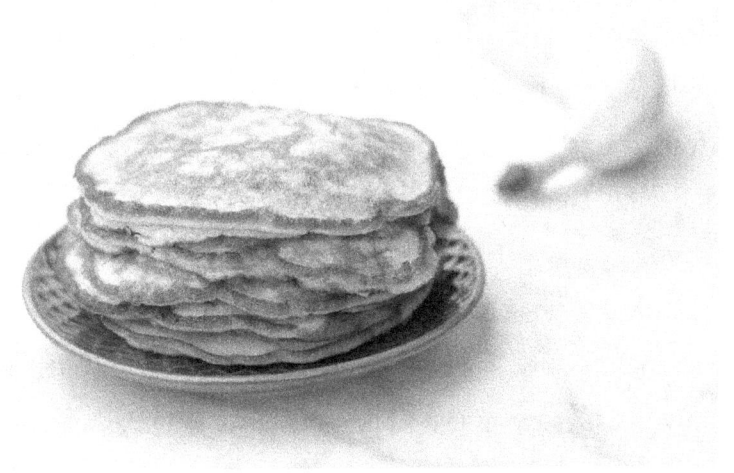

CHAPTER 5

D innertime holds a special place in our daily routine—a time to unwind, connect with loved ones, and indulge in a satisfying meal that nourishes both body and soul. For individuals with PCOS, crafting dinners that not only provide satiety and flavor but also support their health goals is crucial.

In this chapter, we will embark on a culinary journey through a collection of satisfying dinner recipes that prioritize PCOS-friendly ingredients, ensuring that each meal is a delightful and nourishing experience.

Satisfying dinners are more than just a means to satiate hunger; they are an opportunity to incorporate nutrient-rich ingredients, balance macronutrients, and support hormone balance. These recipes have been carefully crafted to offer a variety of options, including seafood, poultry, and vegetarian choices, ensuring that there is something to please every palate.

Picture a dinner where succulent salmon fillets are baked to perfection and served alongside vibrant roasted asparagus and a bed of fluffy quinoa. Or imagine the aromatic aroma of a turmeric-spiced chicken curry simmering on the stovetop, accompanied by cauliflower rice that adds a nutritious twist.

How about indulging in zucchini noodles coated in homemade marinara sauce, topped with flavorful turkey meatballs? Or savoring the stir-fried beef and broccoli with the tantalizing warmth of ginger? These satisfying dinner recipes offer a wealth of flavors and textures that will leave you feeling nourished and satisfied.

Not only are these dinner options delicious, but they also incorporate ingredients known for their beneficial effects on PCOS symptoms. From omega-3 fatty acids found in salmon to the anti-inflammatory properties of turmeric, each recipe has been thoughtfully designed to support your PCOS wellness goals while delivering on taste.

By choosing these satisfying dinner recipes, you are making a conscious decision to prioritize your health and well-being. These meals go beyond mere sustenance; they are a celebration of wholesome ingredients, flavors, and the joy of eating. They offer a moment to slow down, savor each bite, and appreciate the nourishment that comes from food that truly supports your body.

Whether you're cooking for yourself, your family, or friends, these dinner recipes will inspire you to create memorable and nourishing meals that contribute to your overall wellness. Through these culinary adventures, you have the power to embrace the benefits of a PCOS-friendly diet without compromising on taste or satisfaction.

So, let's dive into the realm of satisfying dinners, where wholesome ingredients and delicious flavors combine to create meals that nourish your body and delight your taste buds. With every bite, you are taking a step closer to achieving balance, managing your PCOS symptoms, and embracing the joy of food.

As we embark on this chapter, get ready to savor the delightful flavors, revel in the aromas, and experience the satisfaction of dinners that support your PCOS journey. Let these recipes guide you to create wholesome and gratifying meals that nourish your body and soul.

Now, let's explore the realm of satisfying dinners and discover the delights that await us.

We will explore a collection of delicious and PCOS-friendly dinner recipes that are designed to satiate your hunger, provide essential nutrients, and promote a sense of well-being. From succulent seafood to flavorful poultry and hearty vegetarian options, these recipes will delight your palate while supporting your PCOS wellness goals.

Salmon is a nutritional powerhouse, rich in omega-3 fatty acids and high-quality protein, making it an ideal choice for a PCOS-friendly dinner. To prepare this dish, season the salmon fillets with a blend of herbs and spices, then bake them to perfection.

Serve the salmon alongside roasted asparagus spears and a side of fluffy quinoa, which offers a good dose of fiber and essential minerals. This combination not only creates a visually appealing plate but also provides a well-rounded meal that nourishes your body with heart-healthy fats, vitamins, and minerals.

Turmeric-Spiced Chicken Curry with Cauliflower Rice:
Aromatic and filled with bold flavors, a turmeric-spiced chicken curry is a delightful dinner option. Begin by sautéing onions, garlic, and ginger in a pan, then add boneless chicken pieces and a mixture of fragrant spices, including turmeric, cumin, coriander, and paprika.

Allow the chicken to cook in the flavorful sauce until tender and fully cooked. Serve the curry over a bed of cauliflower rice, which provides a low-carb and nutrient-dense alternative to traditional rice. This dish not only satisfies your taste buds but also incorporates the anti-inflammatory properties of turmeric, supporting your overall wellness.

Zucchini Noodles with Homemade Marinara Sauce and Turkey Meatballs:

For a lighter and vegetable-packed dinner option, zucchini noodles (or "zoodles") with homemade marinara sauce and turkey meatballs are a winning combination. Use a spiralizer to create zucchini noodles, then sauté them briefly in a pan until tender. Prepare a flavorful marinara sauce using fresh tomatoes, herbs, and spices.

Form turkey meatballs seasoned with garlic, onion, and Italian herbs, then bake them until golden and cooked through. Toss the zucchini noodles with the marinara sauce and top with the turkey meatballs for a satisfying and low-carb dinner that's rich in antioxidants, lean protein, and fiber.

Beef Stir-Fry with Broccoli and Ginger:

A beef stir-fry with broccoli and ginger is a quick and easy dinner option that delivers both flavor and nutrition. Begin by stir-frying thinly sliced beef strips in a hot pan until browned and cooked to your liking. Set the beef aside and stir-fry fresh broccoli florets until tender-crisp.

Return the beef to the pan and add a zesty sauce made from soy sauce, ginger, garlic, and a touch of honey for a hint of sweetness. The combination of lean beef, nutrient-rich broccoli, and aromatic ginger creates a satisfying stir-fry that is packed with protein, vitamins, and minerals.

These satisfying dinner recipes offer a diverse array of flavors, textures, and nutrients, ensuring that your evenings are filled with nourishing and delicious meals.

By incorporating these PCOS-friendly dinner options into your routine, you can support your overall well-being, manage symptoms, and enjoy the pleasures of a satisfying and wholesome dinner.

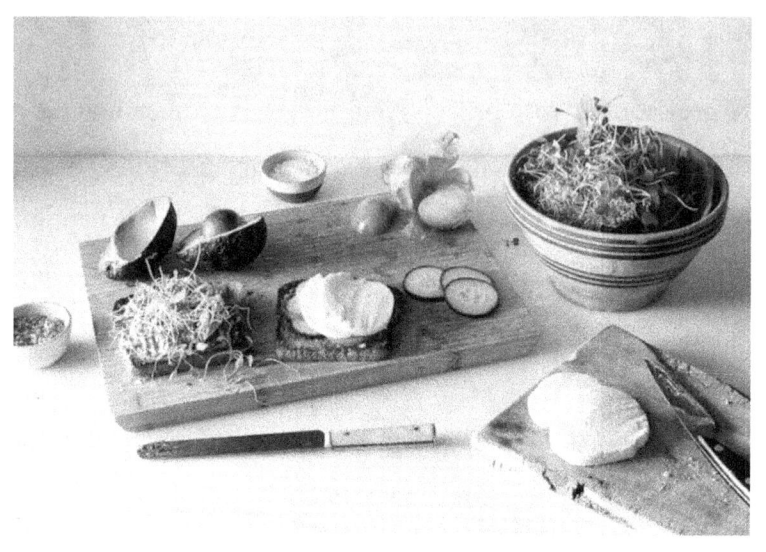

CHAPTER 6

SNACKS AND SMALL BITES

Snacking is an integral part of our daily lives, offering moments of respite and satisfaction between meals. For individuals with PCOS, finding the right snacks that not only satiate cravings but also support their dietary needs can be a challenge.

In this chapter, we will explore a tantalizing array of snacks and small bites specifically designed for PCOS individuals, offering both deliciousness and nourishment in every bite.

Snacks and small bites play a significant role in maintaining stable energy levels, managing hunger, and supporting overall well-being. However, it is essential to choose snacks that align with the nutritional requirements of individuals with PCOS.

The snacks featured in this chapter are carefully crafted to incorporate PCOS-friendly ingredients, striking a balance between flavor, satisfaction, and health.

Imagine the irresistible aroma of roasted chickpeas infused with an enticing blend of herbs and spices, delivering a satisfying crunch and a protein-rich punch. Envision indulging in a creamy avocado hummus, paired with a colorful assortment of vegetable sticks, offering a delectable combination of healthy fats and fiber.

Visualize a refreshing bowl of Greek yogurt adorned with an assortment of mixed berries and a sprinkle of homemade granola, providing a nourishing blend of protein, antioxidants, and crunch. Lastly, picture savoring dark chocolate energy balls, decadently rich and packed with nuts and seeds, delivering a burst of natural sweetness and sustaining energy.

These snacks and small bites are more than just quick treats; they are carefully curated to provide optimal nutrition and support PCOS management.

Each recipe emphasizes nutrient-dense ingredients that promote hormonal balance, stabilize blood sugar levels, and contribute to overall wellness. By choosing these PCOS-friendly snacks, you are not only satisfying your taste buds but also nourishing your body with ingredients that support your health goals.

Snacking should be a mindful and enjoyable experience, allowing you to refuel and rejuvenate throughout the day. By embracing these recipes, you have the opportunity to turn your snack time into a nourishing ritual—a moment to pause, savor, and appreciate the benefits that wholesome ingredients bring to your PCOS wellness journey.

Whether you're seeking a savory, crunchy delight or a sweet, indulgent treat, these snack and small bite recipes offer a diverse range of options to suit your preferences and dietary needs. Each recipe is thoughtfully crafted to provide a balance of macronutrients, incorporating ingredients known for their positive impact on PCOS symptoms.

Incorporating these PCOS-friendly snacks and small bites into your daily routine can help you maintain stable energy levels, manage hunger, and make conscious choices that support your overall well-being. These recipes empower you to snack with intention, taking control of your health while indulging in flavors and textures that satisfy your cravings.

We will explore a variety of delicious and PCOS-friendly snacks and small bites that will not only satisfy your cravings but also provide essential nutrients to keep you energized throughout the day.

Snacks play a vital role in maintaining stable blood sugar levels, managing hunger, and avoiding overindulgence in unhealthy choices.

The snacks featured in this chapter are designed to be nutrient-dense, delicious, and easy to prepare. From crunchy roasted chickpeas to creamy avocado hummus, and from refreshing Greek yogurt with mixed berries to indulgent dark chocolate energy balls, these snack recipes cater to a range of tastes and preferences.

Roasted Chickpeas with Herbs and Spices:

Roasted chickpeas are a fantastic snack option, offering a satisfying crunch along with a boost of protein and fiber. Simply toss cooked chickpeas with a blend of herbs and spices, such as cumin, paprika, garlic powder, and a sprinkle of sea salt. Roast them in the oven until golden and crispy.

These flavorful chickpeas are not only a healthier alternative to processed snacks but also provide essential nutrients and help regulate blood sugar levels.

Creamy Avocado Hummus with Vegetable Sticks:

Hummus is a classic snack, and by adding creamy avocado into the mix, we elevate it to a whole new level. This recipe combines chickpeas, tahini, lemon juice, garlic, and ripe avocado to create a silky and flavorful dip. Pair it with an assortment of fresh vegetable sticks like carrot, cucumber, and bell pepper for a colorful and nutrient-rich snack.

The combination of healthy fats, fiber, and antioxidants makes this snack not only delicious but also beneficial for hormone balance and overall well-being.

Greek Yogurt with Mixed Berries and a Sprinkle of Granola:

Greek yogurt is a versatile and protein-packed snack that can be customized to suit your preferences. Choose a plain, unsweetened Greek yogurt as the base and top it with a medley of mixed berries for a burst of antioxidants and natural sweetness.

Add a sprinkle of homemade granola for a satisfying crunch and additional fiber. This snack not only provides a balance of macronutrients but also supports gut health and satiety.

Dark Chocolate Energy Balls with Nuts and Seeds:

Indulging in a sweet treat doesn't have to derail your PCOS wellness goals. These dark chocolate energy balls are a delightful and nutrient-dense option that satisfies your cravings without compromising on health.

Mix together dates, nuts, seeds, cocoa powder, and a touch of natural sweetener.

Roll the mixture into bite-sized balls and chill them until firm. These energy balls provide a combination of healthy fats, fiber, and antioxidants, making them a guilt-free treat that will keep you energized throughout the day.

These snack and small bite recipes offer a range of flavors, textures, and nutrients, ensuring that you have a variety of options to choose from. By incorporating these PCOS-friendly snacks into your daily routine, you can support stable blood sugar levels, manage hunger, and nourish your body with wholesome ingredients.

Snacking can be an opportunity to infuse your day with nourishment, pleasure, and balance. Let go of the notion that snacking is unhealthy or guilt-inducing, and instead, embrace these recipes as tools to support your overall well-being.

Enjoy the flavors, textures, and benefits that these snacks bring while staying on track with your PCOS journey.

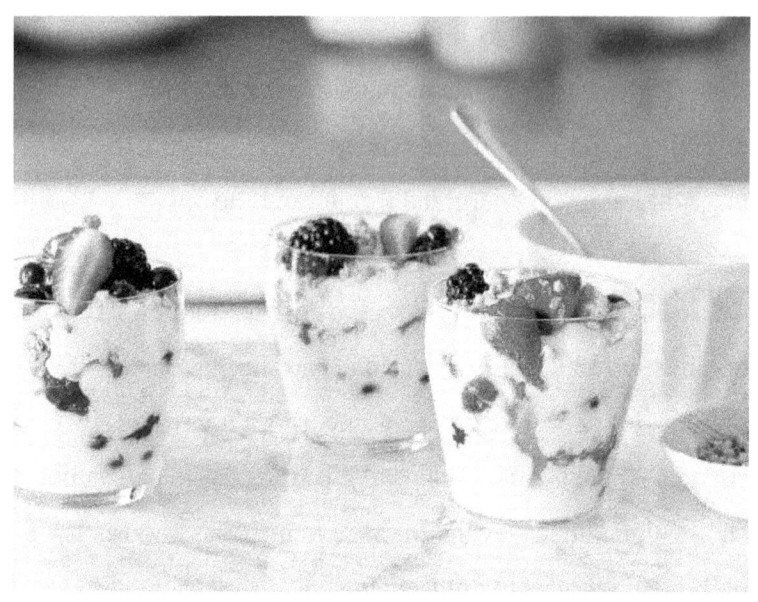

CHAPTER 7

Indulging in sweet treats is a delightful experience that brings joy and satisfaction to our lives. However, for individuals with PCOS, finding sweet treats that align with their dietary needs and support their overall well-being can be a challenge.

The good news is that with the right recipes and ingredients, you can enjoy a wide array of delicious sweet treats that cater to your PCOS wellness goals.

In this chapter, we delve into the realm of sweet treats specifically designed for individuals with PCOS. From guilt-free muffins and creamy puddings to warm baked fruits and wholesome cookies, these recipes will tantalize your taste buds while nourishing your body.

Each recipe is carefully crafted to incorporate PCOS-friendly ingredients that prioritize nutrient-dense choices, blood sugar regulation, and hormonal balance.

When it comes to sweet treats, it's essential to strike a balance between indulgence and health. These recipes offer a perfect harmony of flavors, textures, and nutritional benefits. Whether you're craving the comforting flavors of baked goods or the refreshing creaminess of puddings, this chapter has a variety of options to satisfy your sweet tooth without compromising your PCOS wellness journey.

One of the highlights of this chapter is the gluten-free blueberry muffins made with almond flour. These muffins not only deliver a burst of blueberry goodness but also provide the added benefits of almond flour, which adds a nutty flavor and boosts the protein content.

With natural sweeteners, you can enjoy these moist and fluffy muffins while keeping your blood sugar levels in check.

For those seeking a creamy and nourishing dessert, the coconut milk matcha chia pudding is a must-try. This velvety pudding combines the power of chia seeds, antioxidant-rich matcha powder, and creamy coconut milk. The result is a delightful treat that not only satisfies your cravings but also provides a range of health benefits, including fiber, healthy fats, and antioxidants.

When you're in the mood for a warm and comforting sweet treat, the baked apple slices with cinnamon and almond butter are a perfect choice.

The natural sweetness of the apples, combined with the warmth of cinnamon and the richness of almond butter, creates a delightful combination of flavors. It's a guilt-free dessert that warms your heart and nourishes your body.

Lastly, the banana and walnut oat cookies offer a wholesome option for satisfying your sweet cravings. Mashed bananas, oats, chopped walnuts, and a touch of natural sweetener come together to create chewy and satisfying cookies.

These treats strike the perfect balance between sweetness and nutrition, providing you with carbohydrates, healthy fats, and fiber to support your PCOS wellness.

With these sweet treat recipes at your disposal, you can indulge in the pleasure of desserts while prioritizing your PCOS management. Each recipe invites you to savor the flavors, enjoy the textures, and embrace the joy of sweet treats that nourish your body and contribute to hormonal balance.

We will explore a delectable collection of sweet treats specifically designed for individuals with PCOS. From gluten-free blueberry muffins with almond flour to coconut milk matcha chia pudding, and from baked apple slices with cinnamon and almond butter to banana and walnut oat cookies, these recipes will satisfy your cravings while keeping your PCOS wellness in mind.

Gluten-Free Blueberry Muffins with Almond Flour:

Start your sweet journey with these irresistible gluten-free blueberry muffins made with almond flour. Not only are they fluffy and bursting with juicy blueberries, but they are also a healthier alternative to traditional muffins.

Almond flour adds a nutty flavor and a boost of protein, while natural sweeteners like honey or maple syrup provide just the right amount of sweetness. Enjoy these moist and flavorful muffins without compromising on your PCOS wellness goals.

Coconut Milk Matcha Chia Pudding:

For a creamy and refreshing sweet treat, dive into a bowl of coconut milk matcha chia pudding. This velvety pudding combines the goodness of chia seeds, antioxidant-rich matcha powder, and creamy coconut milk. The result is a luscious and nutrient-packed dessert that not only satisfies your cravings but also provides a range of health benefits.

The combination of chia seeds, matcha, and coconut milk offers a generous dose of healthy fats, fiber, and antioxidants, making this pudding a perfect addition to your PCOS-friendly repertoire.

Baked Apple Slices with Cinnamon and Almond Butter:

When you're in the mood for a warm and comforting sweet treat, look no further than baked apple slices with cinnamon and almond butter. This simple yet satisfying dessert combines the natural sweetness of apples with the warmth of cinnamon and the richness of almond butter.

By baking the apple slices until tender, you release their natural flavors and create a delightful treat that is both comforting and nourishing. Enjoy the cozy aroma and the delightful combination of flavors as you savor this guilt-free dessert.

Indulge in the goodness of these banana and walnut oat cookies that are not only delicious but also packed with wholesome ingredients. Mashed bananas, oats, chopped walnuts, and a touch of natural sweetener come together to create chewy and satisfying cookies.

These cookies offer a balance of carbohydrates, healthy fats, and fiber, making them a guilt-free option for satisfying your sweet cravings. Enjoy them as a snack or as a dessert, knowing that you are nourishing your body while satisfying your taste buds.

These sweet treat recipes are thoughtfully crafted to provide you with options that are both delicious and supportive of your PCOS wellness journey. They allow you to enjoy the pleasure of desserts without compromising on your health goals. By incorporating these recipes into your lifestyle, you can indulge in the flavors and textures you love while nourishing your body with PCOS-friendly ingredients.

Take a moment to explore the recipes in this chapter and discover a world of sweet delights that contribute to your overall well-being. These treats are designed to bring joy to your taste buds while supporting your PCOS management.

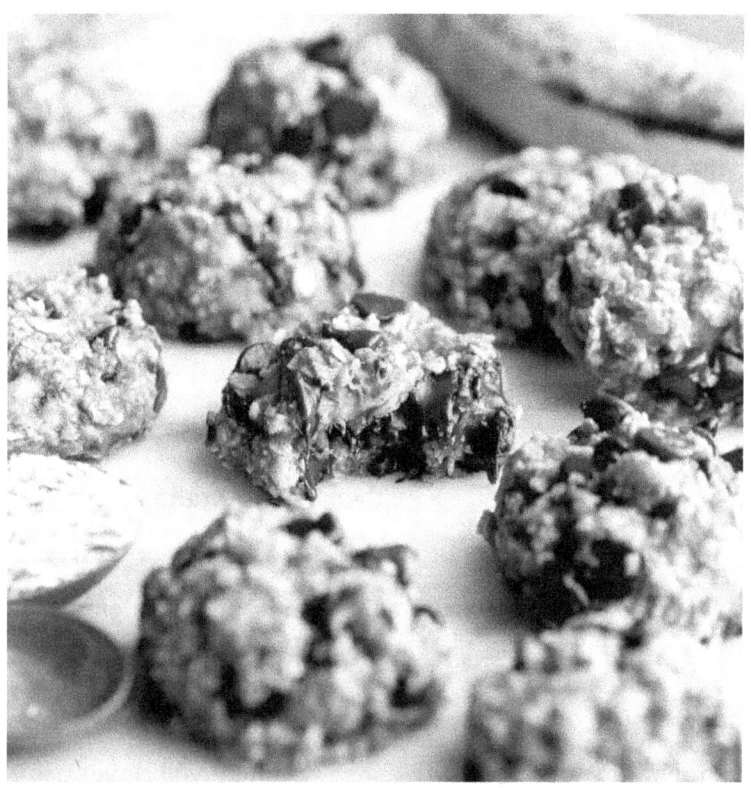

CHAPTER 8

Meal planning is a valuable tool in maintaining a healthy lifestyle, and it becomes even more crucial when managing a condition like Polycystic Ovary Syndrome (PCOS). By proactively organizing your meals and considering the nutritional needs associated with PCOS, you can ensure that you're nourishing your body with the right foods and supporting your overall well-being.

We will dives into the practical aspects of meal planning, equipping you with effective strategies to make the process efficient, enjoyable, and PCOS-friendly. Additionally, it offers valuable guidance on navigating the grocery store and stocking your pantry with nutritious ingredients that align with your dietary goals.

This chapter explores various facets of meal planning, emphasizing the importance of customization, organization, and smart decision-making. From setting goals to utilizing leftovers, you'll discover a range of strategies to streamline your meal planning routine and make it an integral part of your PCOS management journey.

In addition to meal planning, this chapter also provides essential tips for shopping with PCOS in mind. It offers insights on how to navigate the grocery store, make informed choices, and build a well-stocked pantry filled with PCOS-friendly ingredients. By understanding the foundations of effective meal planning and smart shopping, you can take control of your nutrition and support your PCOS wellness goals.

Whether you're new to meal planning or looking to enhance your existing approach, Chapter 8 is your comprehensive guide. It empowers you with practical knowledge, actionable tips, and real-life strategies to transform your meal planning experience and optimize your food choices for PCOS management.

By investing time and effort into meal planning and adopting smart shopping practices, you can create a solid foundation for your PCOS wellness journey. This chapter will inspire and guide you, offering valuable insights and empowering you to make informed decisions when it comes to nourishing your body with wholesome and PCOS-friendly foods.

Get ready to embark on a transformative journey of meal planning and shopping, armed with the knowledge and tools to make nourishing choices that support your overall health and well-being. Let Chapter 8 be your trusted resource as you explore the world of PCOS-centric meal planning and shopping tips, and discover the positive impact it can have on your life.

We will explore effective meal planning techniques, stocking your pantry with PCOS-friendly ingredients, navigating the grocery store with a PCOS shopping guide, and tips for staying organized and on track with your meal planning efforts.

10 Strategies for Meal Planning with PCOS in Mind:

1. Set Goals:

To start your meal planning journey, it's important to establish clear goals for managing your PCOS. These goals can vary from person to person and may include weight management, blood sugar control, hormone regulation, or addressing specific PCOS symptoms.

Consulting with your healthcare provider or a registered dietitian can provide valuable insights and recommendations tailored to your individual needs.

2. Create a Meal Planning Schedule:

Allocate dedicated time each week for meal planning. Choose a day that works best for you, taking into account your schedule and availability.

Make meal planning a regular routine to ensure consistency and make the process more efficient. This will help you stay on track with your PCOS-friendly eating plan.

3. Assess Your Needs:

Take some time to assess your dietary preferences, food restrictions, and any challenges you may face due to PCOS. Consider factors such as insulin resistance, hormonal imbalances, or weight concerns when planning your meals. This will help you create a meal plan that addresses your specific needs and supports your overall health.

4. Emphasize Balanced Nutrition:

Prioritize a well-rounded diet that includes a variety of nutrient-dense foods. Focus on incorporating whole grains, lean proteins, healthy fats, and an abundance of fruits and vegetables into your meals.

Be mindful of the specific nutritional needs associated with PCOS and consider including foods that are known to support PCOS management, such as flaxseeds, cinnamon, turmeric, and leafy greens.

5. Incorporate Portion Control: Pay attention to portion sizes to maintain a healthy weight and support insulin sensitivity. Measuring tools, such as cups and scales, can help ensure accurate portioning.

Aim for a balanced plate that includes appropriate portions of proteins, carbohydrates, and fats to provide essential nutrients and support your PCOS management goals.

6. Plan for Regular Meals and Snacks:
Structure your meal plan to include three main meals and two to three snacks throughout the day. This helps maintain steady energy levels, stabilizes blood sugar levels, and prevents overeating.

Choose nutrient-dense snacks that provide sustained energy and support your PCOS management. Incorporate a combination of protein, healthy fats, and fiber-rich carbohydrates in your snacks.

7. Batch Cooking and Meal Prep:
Batch cooking involves preparing larger quantities of food at once, which can save time and ensure you have healthy options readily available.

Cook large batches of grains, proteins, and vegetables that can be incorporated into multiple meals throughout the week. Portion and store them in individual containers for easy meal prep and quick grab-and-go options.

8. Use Meal Templates:

Meal templates provide a helpful framework for planning your meals. Create a template for each meal category, such as breakfast, lunch, dinner, and snacks.

Include a variety of food groups in each template to ensure balanced nutrition. This ensures that you're getting a mix of macronutrients (carbohydrates, proteins, and fats) and micronutrients (vitamins and minerals) in your meals.

9. Utilize Leftovers:

Make the most of leftovers by recycling them into new meals. This helps reduce food waste and saves time and effort in meal preparation.

For example, you can transform cooked proteins and vegetables into salads, wraps, or stir-fries for the next day's meal. Get creative with your leftovers to keep your meals interesting and diverse.

10. Stay Flexible and Adapt:

Remember that meal planning is a flexible process. Be open to adjustments and modifications based on your evolving needs, preferences, and lifestyle.

Experiment with new recipes, flavors, and ingredients to keep mealtime exciting and enjoyable. Listen to your body's cues and make changes accordingly to support your overall well-being.

By following these strategies for meal planning with PCOS in mind, you can create a personalized approach that caters specifically to your PCOS management needs. It allows you to prioritize balanced nutrition, portion control, and flexibility, ultimately supporting your overall health and wellness.

How to Stock Your Pantry with PCOS-Friendly Ingredients:

Stocking your pantry with PCOS-friendly ingredients is a key aspect of maintaining a healthy and supportive diet. By keeping your pantry well-stocked with nutritious options, you can easily create nourishing meals and snacks that align with your PCOS management goals.

In this section, we will explore essential tips and recommendations for stocking your pantry with PCOS-friendly ingredients.

Whole Grains:

Whole grains are an excellent source of fiber and provide sustained energy. Opt for options like brown rice, quinoa, oats, and whole wheat pasta or bread.

These grains have a lower glycemic index, which means they release sugar into the bloodstream more slowly, helping to stabilize blood sugar levels.

Lean Proteins:

Protein is an important nutrient for managing PCOS. Stock your pantry with lean protein sources such as skinless chicken breast, turkey, fish, tofu, and legumes like lentils and chickpeas.

Incorporating protein into your meals helps promote satiety, regulate blood sugar levels, and support healthy weight management.

Healthy Fats:

Include heart-healthy fats in your pantry. Opt for sources like olive oil, avocado oil, nuts (almonds, walnuts, cashews), seeds (flaxseeds, chia seeds), and nut butter (almond butter, peanut butter).

These fats provide essential fatty acids and help promote hormone balance and reduce inflammation in the body.

Fresh and Frozen Produce:

Keep a variety of fresh and frozen fruits and vegetables on hand. Choose colorful options like berries, leafy greens, broccoli, cauliflower, bell peppers, and sweet potatoes.

Fresh produce can be used for salads, snacks, and cooking, while frozen options are convenient for smoothies, stir-fries, and soups.

They retain their nutrients and offer versatility in meal preparation.

Herbs and Spices:

Enhance the flavor of your meals with herbs and spices. Stock up on essentials like cinnamon, turmeric, ginger, garlic powder, oregano, basil, and paprika.

These seasonings add depth and aroma to your dishes without relying on excess salt, sugar, or unhealthy condiments.

Canned Goods:

Choose canned goods with minimal additives and sodium. Opt for options like canned beans (black beans, chickpeas), diced tomatoes, and canned fish (tuna, salmon).

Canned goods provide convenience and versatility, making them useful for creating quick and nutritious meals.

PCOS-Supportive Ingredients:

Consider incorporating specific ingredients known for their benefits in managing PCOS symptoms. Examples include flaxseeds (rich in omega-3 fatty acids), cinnamon (helps regulate blood sugar), and green tea (contains antioxidants).

These ingredients can be used in various recipes and can contribute to the overall support of your PCOS management goals.

Non-Dairy Milk Alternatives:

If you prefer non-dairy milk, stock your pantry with options like almond milk, coconut milk, or oat milk. Ensure you choose unsweetened varieties to avoid added sugars.

Non-dairy milk alternatives can be used in smoothies, baking, and as a dairy substitute in various recipes.

Healthy Snack Options:

Keep a selection of PCOS-friendly snacks in your pantry. This can include nuts, seeds, dried fruits (in moderation), low-sugar granola bars, and dark chocolate (70% cocoa or higher).These snacks provide a balance of nutrients, satisfy cravings, and offer healthier alternatives to processed snacks.

Low-Sugar Condiments:

Opt for low-sugar condiments to add flavor to your meals. Choose options like mustard, hot sauce, apple cider vinegar, and low-sodium soy sauce.

These condiments can add tang and spice to your dishes without adding excessive sugars or unhealthy additives.

By stocking your pantry with these PCOS-friendly ingredients, you will have a solid foundation for creating wholesome meals that support your PCOS management goals.

Regularly check your pantry and restock items as needed to ensure you always have the necessary ingredients on hand. With a well-stocked pantry, you can approach meal preparation with confidence and make nourishing choices that contribute to your overall well-being.

Navigating the Grocery Store: PCOS Shopping Guide:

Navigating the grocery store with a focus on PCOS-friendly foods is an essential skill for managing your condition and making informed choices.

The following PCOS shopping guide will provide you with valuable tips and strategies to help you navigate the aisles and select the best options for your health and wellness.

Prepare a Shopping List:

Before heading to the grocery store, create a shopping list based on your meal plan and nutritional goals.

Having a list will help you stay focused and prevent impulse buying of unhealthy or unnecessary items.

Shop the Perimeter:

The perimeter of the grocery store is typically where you'll find fresh produce, lean proteins, dairy, and whole foods.

Aim to spend the majority of your time in these sections, as they offer the most nutrient-dense options.

Read Food Labels:

Become familiar with reading food labels to make informed choices. Pay attention to serving sizes, sugar content, and the presence of artificial additives or preservatives.

Look for products with minimal ingredients and avoid those with high amounts of added sugars, unhealthy fats, or artificial sweeteners.

Choose Whole Foods:

Opt for whole foods whenever possible. These are foods that are minimally processed and retain their natural nutrients.

Focus on fresh fruits and vegetables, lean meats, whole grains, and legumes. These foods provide essential vitamins, minerals, and fiber.

Be Mindful of Carbohydrates:
Carbohydrates can significantly impact blood sugar levels. Choose complex carbohydrates that are high in fiber and have a lower glycemic index.
Opt for whole grains, legumes, and non-starchy vegetables over refined grains, sugary snacks, and processed foods.

Prioritize Lean Proteins:
Protein is important for managing PCOS symptoms and promoting satiety. Choose lean sources such as skinless poultry, fish, tofu, and legumes.
Avoid processed meats that may contain additives and unhealthy fats.

Include Healthy Fats:
Incorporate healthy fats into your shopping cart. Look for sources like avocados, nuts, seeds, and cold-pressed oils.

Avoid trans fats and limit your intake of saturated fats, which can contribute to inflammation and hormonal imbalance.

Minimize Processed Foods:

Processed foods are often high in refined sugars, unhealthy fats, and additives. Limit your consumption of packaged snacks, sugary beverages, and pre-packaged meals.

Instead, focus on whole, nutrient-dense foods to support your PCOS management goals.

Consider Organic and Locally Sourced Options:

If feasible, choose organic and locally sourced products, especially for fruits and vegetables that are known to have higher pesticide residues.

Organic options can reduce your exposure to potentially harmful chemicals and support sustainable farming practices.

Don't Shop on an Empty Stomach:

Shopping on an empty stomach can lead to impulse buying and choosing less healthy options.

Eat a balanced meal or snack before heading to the grocery store to make more mindful choices.

Plan for Meal Prep:

Consider purchasing containers, storage bags, and other meal prep essentials to help you prepare and store meals in advance.

Meal prepping can save time, reduce stress, and ensure that you have nourishing meals readily available.

Stay Mindful of Portion Sizes:

Even when choosing healthy options, be mindful of portion sizes to maintain a balanced diet.

Use measuring cups, food scales, or visual references to guide portion control.

Navigating the grocery store with a PCOS shopping guide empowers you to make choices that support your health and well-being. By selecting nutrient-dense whole foods, reading labels

Staying organized and on track with your PCOS-friendly meal plan is crucial for maintaining a healthy diet and managing your symptoms effectively.

The following tips will help you stay organized, stay motivated, and stay on track with your PCOS wellness journey:

1. Create a Weekly Meal Plan:

Set aside some time each week to plan your meals and snacks in advance. This will help you stay focused, avoid impulsive food choices, and ensure you have all the necessary ingredients on hand.

Consider using a meal planning template or app to streamline the process and make it easier to stick to your plan.

2. Prepare a Shopping List:

Based on your weekly meal plan, create a detailed shopping list of all the ingredients you'll need.

Having a shopping list will prevent you from forgetting key items and reduce the temptation to buy unhealthy foods.

3. Batch Cooking and Meal Prepping:
Dedicate a specific day or time each week for batch cooking and meal prepping.

Prepare large batches of staple foods such as grains, proteins, and vegetables that can be used in multiple meals throughout the week. Portion out meals and snacks into individual containers for easy grab-and-go options.

4. Use Food Storage Containers:
Invest in a variety of food storage containers in different sizes and shapes to keep your meals organized and fresh.

Label containers with the meal or snack name and date to help you stay organized and prevent food waste.

5. Portion Control:
Practice portion control by using measuring cups, food scales, or visual cues to ensure you're consuming appropriate portion sizes.

This will help you maintain a balanced diet and prevent overeating.

6. Schedule Regular Eating Times:
Establish a routine by scheduling regular eating times throughout the day.
Eating at consistent intervals can help regulate your blood sugar levels and prevent unhealthy snacking or excessive hunger.

7. Set Realistic Goals:
Set realistic and achievable goals for yourself. Break them down into smaller milestones to stay motivated and track your progress.
Celebrate your victories along the road to preserve a good outlook.

8. Keep a Food Journal:
Consider keeping a food journal to track your meals, snacks, and any symptoms or changes you experience.
This can help you identify patterns, trigger foods, and areas for improvement in your diet.

9. Stay Hydrated:

Don't forget to prioritize hydration. Keep a water bottle with you at all times and set notes to drink water throughout the day.

Staying hydrated supports digestion, metabolism, and overall health.

10. Practice Self-Care:

Remember to prioritize self-care in your routine. Manage stress levels, get enough sleep, engage in physical activity, and take time for activities you enjoy.

A well-balanced and happy lifestyle is key to maintaining a healthy diet.

By implementing these tips for staying organized and on track, you'll be better equipped to stick to your PCOS-friendly meal plan, make healthy choices, and manage your symptoms effectively. Remember that consistency and mindfulness are key to long-term success.

By mastering the art of meal planning and smart grocery shopping, you can take control of your PCOS management and nourish your body with balanced and satisfying meals.

With careful consideration of your dietary needs, stocking your pantry with PCOS-friendly ingredients, making informed choices at the grocery store, and staying organized and on track, you can create a supportive environment that facilitates your journey towards better health.

BONUS

E mbark on a transformative journey towards optimal health and well-being with the 4 Weeks PCOS Meal Planner Timetable. This comprehensive guide is your roadmap to balanced meals, nutrient-rich ingredients, and PCOS-friendly recipes carefully designed to support your unique needs.

Say goodbye to uncertainty and hello to a structured meal plan that simplifies your life, nourishes your body, and empowers you on your PCOS wellness journey. With four weeks of delicious recipes and expert guidance, this meal planner is your key to reclaiming control over your health and embracing a vibrant, fulfilling life. Let the journey begin.

WEEK 1 MEAL PLANNER

	BREAKFAST	LUNCH	DINNER	SNACKS
MON	Spinach and Mushroom Omelette	Quinoa and Roasted Vegetable Salad with Lemon-Tahini Dressing	Baked Salmon with Roasted Asparagus and Quinoa	Greek Yogurt with Mixed Berries
TUE	Overnight Chia Pudding with Fresh Fruits	Grilled Chicken and Avocado Lettuce Wraps	Turmeric-Spiced Chicken Curry with Cauliflower Rice	Celery Sticks with Almond Butter
WED	Fluffy Gluten-Free Pancakes with Berry Compote	Sweet Potato and Black Bean Chili	Zucchini Noodles with Homemade Marinara Sauce and Turkey Meatballs	Roasted Chickpeas with Herbs and Spices
THUR	Green Smoothie with Spinach, Banana, and Almond Milk	Mediterranean-Style Tuna Salad with Greek Yogurt Dressing	Beef Stir-Fry with Broccoli and Ginger	Creamy Avocado Hummus with Vegetable Sticks
FRI	Scrambled Eggs with Sautéed Vegetables	Quinoa Salad with Grilled Shrimp and Citrus Dressing	Baked Chicken Breast with Roasted Brussels Sprouts and Quinoa	Cottage Cheese with Sliced Peaches
SAT	Veggie-Packed Frittata with Herbs and Feta	Lentil Soup with a Side of Mixed Greens Salad	Spaghetti Squash with Turkey Bolognese Sauce	Greek Yogurt with a Drizzle of Honey
SUN	Avocado Toast on Whole Grain Bread	Chickpea Salad with Lemon-Tahini Dressing	Grilled Salmon with Quinoa and Steamed Broccoli	Cucumber Slices with Tzatziki Sauce

I CAN DO IT

WEEK 2 MEAL PLANNER

	BREAKFAST	LUNCH	DINNER	SNACKS
MON	Green Smoothie Bowl with Spinach, Banana, and Almond Milk, topped with	Grilled Chicken Salad with Mixed Greens, Cherry Tomatoes, Cucumbers, and Balsamic Vinaigrette	Baked Cod with Lemon-Herb Quinoa and Steamed Broccoli	Greek Yogurt with Sliced Almonds and a drizzle of Honey
TUE	Scrambled Eggs with Spinach, Bell Peppers, and Feta Cheese	Quinoa and Black Bean Stuffed Bell Peppers, served with a side of Mixed Greens	Turkey Meatball Lettuce Wraps with Zucchini Noodles	Apple Slices with Almond Butter
WED	Overnight Chia Pudding with Almond Milk, topped with Fresh Berries and a sprinkle of Chia Seeds	Mediterranean Quinoa Salad with Grilled Shrimp, Tomatoes, Cucumbers, Kalamata Olives, and Feta Cheese	Chicken Stir-Fry with Broccoli, Bell Peppers, and Snow Peas, served over Cauliflower Rice	Veggie Sticks with Creamy Avocado Hummus
THUR	Gluten-Free Banana Pancakes with a drizzle of Maple Syrup	Lentil Soup with a side of Mixed Greens Salad	Baked Salmon with Roasted Asparagus and Quinoa	Greek Yogurt with Mixed Berries and a sprinkle of Granola
FRI	Vegetable Omelette with Spinach, Mushrooms, Bell Peppers, and Goat Cheese	Chickpea Salad with Lemon-Tahini Dressing, served over a bed of Mixed Greens	Beef Stir-Fry with Broccoli, Snap Peas, and Sesame Ginger Sauce, served over Brown Rice	Cottage Cheese with Sliced Peaches
SAT	Avocado Toast on Whole Grain Bread, topped with Sliced Tomatoes and a sprinkle of Everything Bagel Seasoning	Quinoa and Roasted Vegetable Salad with Lemon-Tahini Dressing	Spaghetti Squash with Turkey Bolognese Sauce	Cherry Tomatoes with Mozzarella Cheese
SUN	Smoothie Bowl with Acai, Mixed Berries, Banana, and Almond Milk, topped with Coconut Flakes and Chia Seeds	Grilled Chicken and Avocado Wrap with Lettuce, Tomato, and Greek Yogurt Dressing	Baked Chicken Breast with Roasted Brussels Sprouts and Quinoa	Cucumber Slices with Tzatziki Sauce

I CAN DO IT

WEEK 3 MEAL PLANNER

	BREAKFAST	LUNCH	DINNER	SNACKS
MON	Spinach and Mushroom Omelette with Goat Cheese	Quinoa Salad with Roasted Butternut Squash, Cranberries, and Pumpkin Seeds	Baked Herb-Roasted Chicken Thighs with Steamed Green Beans and Quinoa	Sliced Bell Peppers with Hummus
TUE	Blueberry Protein Smoothie with Greek Yogurt and Almond Milk	Greek Salad with Grilled Chicken, Cucumbers, Tomatoes, Olives, and Feta Cheese	Zucchini Noodles with Turkey Meatballs and Homemade Marinara Sauce	Roasted Chickpeas with Turmeric
WED	Overnight Chia Pudding with Coconut Milk, topped with Fresh Berries and a sprinkle of Coconut Flakes	Lentil Soup with a side of Mixed Greens Salad	Grilled Salmon with Lemon-Dill Sauce, served with Roasted Brussels Sprouts and Quinoa	Mixed Nuts and Dried Fruit
THUR	Gluten-Free Banana Pancakes with a drizzle of Maple Syrup	Quinoa and Black Bean Burrito Bowl with Avocado, Salsa, and Greek Yogurt	Baked Cod with Roasted Asparagus and Brown Rice	Greek Yogurt with Mixed Berries and a sprinkle of Granola
FRI	Veggie Scramble with Spinach, Bell Peppers, Mushrooms, and Feta Cheese	Chickpea Salad with Lemon-Tahini Dressing, served over a bed of Mixed Greens	Beef Stir-Fry with Broccoli, Snap Peas, and Sesame Ginger Sauce, served over Brown Rice	Rice Cakes with Almond Butter
SAT	Avocado Toast on Whole Grain Bread, topped with Sliced Tomatoes and a sprinkle of Everything Bagel Seasoning	Quinoa and Roasted Vegetable Salad with Lemon-Tahini Dressing	Baked Chicken Breast with Roasted Brussels Sprouts and Quinoa	Greek Yogurt with a drizzle of Honey
SUN	Green Smoothie Bowl with Spinach, Pineapple, and Almond Milk, topped with Fresh Berries and Granola	Grilled Chicken and Avocado Wrap with Lettuce, Tomato, and Greek Yogurt Dressing	Baked Salmon with Quinoa Pilaf and Steamed Broccoli	Cucumber Slices with Tzatziki Sauce

I CAN DO IT

WEEK 4 MEAL PLANNER

	BREAKFAST	LUNCH	DINNER	SNACKS
MON	Veggie Omelette with Spinach, Bell Peppers, and Feta Cheese	Mediterranean-style Quinoa Salad with Cherry Tomatoes, Cucumber, Kalamata Olives, and Feta Cheese	Grilled Shrimp Skewers with Quinoa Tabbouleh and Grilled Zucchini	Greek Yogurt with Sliced Almonds and a sprinkle of Cinnamon
TUE	Blueberry Protein Smoothie with Greek Yogurt and Almond Milk	Chicken and Vegetable Stir-Fry with Brown Rice	Baked Herb-Roasted Chicken Breast with Steamed Broccoli and Quinoa	Carrot Sticks with Hummus
WED	Overnight Chia Pudding with Coconut Milk, topped with Fresh Berries and a sprinkle of Coconut Flakes	Lentil Soup with a side of Mixed Greens Salad	Zucchini Noodles with Turkey Meatballs and Homemade Marinara Sauce	Mixed Nuts and Dried Fruit
THUR	Gluten-Free Banana Pancakes with a drizzle of Maple Syrup	Chickpea Salad with Lemon-Tahini Dressing, served over a bed of Mixed Greens	Baked Cod with Roasted Asparagus and Quinoa	Rice Cakes with Almond Butter
FRI	Veggie Scramble with Spinach, Bell Peppers, Mushrooms, and Feta Cheese	Quinoa and Black Bean Burrito Bowl with Avocado, Salsa, and Greek Yogurt	Beef Stir-Fry with Broccoli, Snap Peas, and Sesame Ginger Sauce, served over Brown Rice	Greek Yogurt with a drizzle of Honey
SAT	Avocado Toast on Whole Grain Bread, topped with Sliced Tomatoes and a sprinkle of Everything Bagel Seasoning	Quinoa and Roasted Vegetable Salad with Lemon-Tahini Dressing	Baked Chicken Breast with Roasted Brussels Sprouts and Quinoa	Cherry Tomatoes with Mozzarella Cheese
SUN	Green Smoothie Bowl with Spinach, Pineapple, and Almond Milk, topped with Fresh Berries and Granola	Grilled Chicken and Avocado Wrap with Lettuce, Tomato, and Greek Yogurt Dressing	Baked Salmon with Quinoa Pilaf and Steamed Broccoli	Cucumber Slices with Tzatziki Sauce

I CAN DO IT

20 Powerful Recipes for PCOS

Unlock the power of culinary healing with "20 Powerful Recipes for PCOS." This collection of carefully curated recipes is your gateway to nourishing your body, balancing hormones, and embracing optimal health.

Each recipe is thoughtfully crafted with PCOS individuals in mind, incorporating nutrient-rich ingredients and flavors that tantalize the taste buds. From vibrant smoothie bowls to satisfying main courses and decadent desserts, these recipes empower you to take charge of your well-being.

Discover the transformative potential of foods that support hormone balance, boost energy levels, and promote overall wellness. With "20 Powerful Recipes for PCOS," you have the tools to create a delicious and empowering culinary journey that will revolutionize your relationship with food and help you thrive with PCOS.

20 RECIPES

Let these recipes be your guide on the path to vibrant health and self-discovery.

Recipes

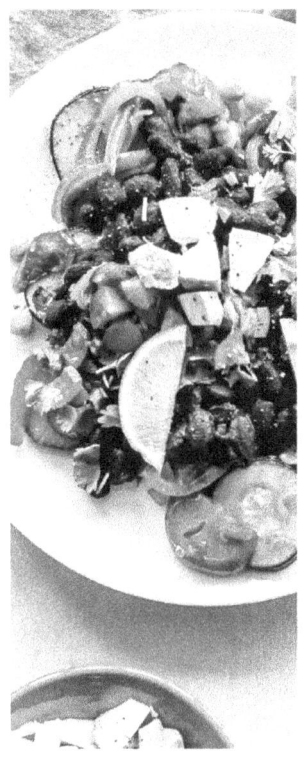

Veggie Omelette with Spinach, Bell Peppers, and Feta Cheese

INGREDIENT

- 2 eggs
- 1 cup fresh spinach leaves
- 1/4 cup diced bell peppers
- 2 tablespoons crumbled feta cheese
- Salt and pepper to taste
- Cooking spray or olive oil for cooking

PREPARATION

- In a bowl, whisk the eggs until well beaten.
- Heat a non-stick skillet over medium heat and lightly coat with cooking spray or olive oil.
- Add the diced bell peppers and sauté for a few minutes until slightly softened.
- Add the spinach leaves and cook until wilted.
- Pour the beaten eggs into the skillet over the vegetables.
- Cook the omelette until the edges start to set, then gently lift and fold the omelette in half.
- Sprinkle the crumbled feta cheese on top and cook for another minute or until the eggs are fully cooked and the cheese is melted.
- Season with salt and pepper to taste.
- Serve hot and enjoy!

Veggie Omelette with Spinach, Bell Peppers, and Feta Cheese

INGREDIENT

- 1 cup mixed berries (strawberries, blueberries, raspberries)
- 1/2 cup Greek yogurt
- 1/2 cup almond milk (or any non-dairy milk)
- 1 tablespoon honey (optional)
- Ice cubes

PREPARATION

- In a blender, combine the mixed berries, Greek yogurt, almond milk, and honey (if desired).
- Add a handful of ice cubes to the blender.
- Blend until smooth and creamy.
- Pour into a glass and enjoy the refreshing mixed berry smoothie.

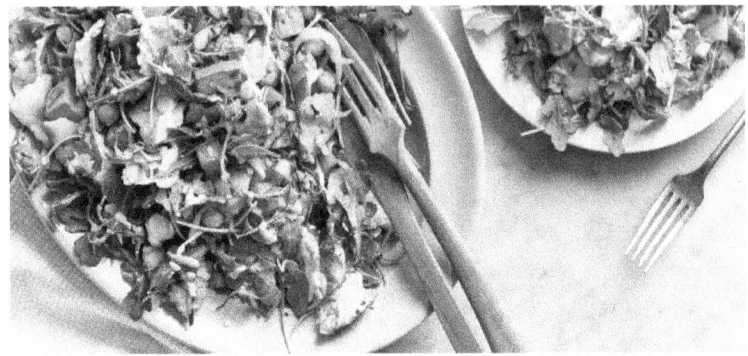

Baked Salmon with Roasted Asparagus and Quinoa

INGREDIENT

- 4 salmon fillets
- 1 bunch asparagus, trimmed
- 2 tablespoons olive oil
- 1 teaspoon lemon zest
- Salt and pepper to taste
- 1 cup cooked quinoa
- Fresh lemon wedges for serving

PREPARATION

- Preheat the oven to 400°F (200°C).
- Place the salmon fillets on a baking sheet lined with parchment paper.
- Drizzle with olive oil and sprinkle with lemon zest, salt, and pepper.
- Arrange the trimmed asparagus around the salmon fillets on the baking sheet.
- Drizzle the asparagus with olive oil and season with salt and pepper.
- Bake in the preheated oven for about 12-15 minutes or until the salmon is cooked through and the asparagus is tender.
- While the salmon and asparagus are baking, prepare the quinoa according to package instructions.
- Serve the baked salmon and roasted asparagus alongside the cooked quinoa.
- Squeeze fresh lemon juice over the salmon fillets before serving.

Quinoa Salad with Roasted Vegetables and Lemon-Tahini Dressing

INGREDIENT

- 1 cup cooked quinoa
- 1 cup mixed roasted vegetables (such as bell peppers, zucchini, eggplant, and cherry tomatoes)
- 2 tablespoons chopped fresh herbs (such as parsley, basil, or mint)
- 2 tablespoons lemon-tahini dressing (see recipe below)

PREPARATION

- Cook quinoa according to package instructions and let it cool.
- Preheat the oven to 400°F (200°C).
- Toss the mixed vegetables with a drizzle of olive oil, salt, and pepper.
- Spread the vegetables on a baking sheet and roast in the preheated oven for about 20 minutes or until tender.
- In a bowl, combine the cooked quinoa, roasted vegetables, and chopped fresh herbs.
- Drizzle with lemon-tahini dressing and toss to coat evenly.
- Serve the quinoa salad as a refreshing and nutritious lunch option.

Greek Yogurt with Mixed Berries and
a sprinkle of Chia Seeds

INGREDIENT

- 1/2 cup Greek yogurt
- 1/2 cup mixed berries (such as strawberries, blueberries, and raspberries)
- 1 teaspoon chia seeds

PREPARATION

- In a bowl, scoop the Greek yogurt.
- Top with the mixed berries and sprinkle with chia seeds.
- Mix lightly to combine.
- Enjoy the creamy and tangy Greek yogurt with the burst of flavors from the mixed berries and the added crunch of chia seeds.

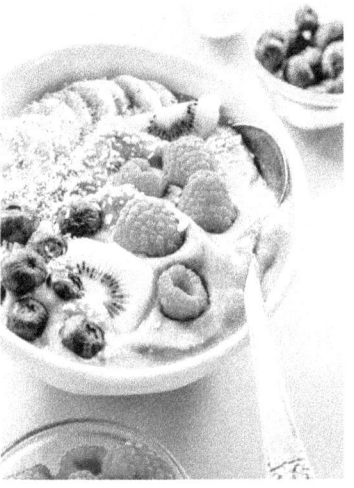

Green Smoothie Bowl with Spinach,
Pineapple, and Almond Milk, topped
with Fresh Berries and Granola

INGREDIENT

- 1 frozen banana
- 1 cup fresh spinach
- 1/2 cup pineapple chunks (fresh or frozen)
- 1/2 cup unsweetened almond milk (or any other plant-based milk)
- 1 tablespoon almond butter
- Toppings: fresh berries (such as strawberries, blueberries, raspberries), granola, shredded coconut

PREPARATION

- In a blender, combine the frozen banana, fresh spinach, pineapple chunks, almond milk, and almond butter.
- Blend on high speed until smooth and creamy. If needed, add more almond milk to achieve the desired consistency.
- Pour the green smoothie into a bowl.
- Arrange the toppings on the smoothie, such as fresh berries, granola, and shredded coconut.
- Serve the green smoothie bowl immediately and enjoy it as a refreshing and nutritious breakfast or snack.

Grilled Chicken and
Avocado Lettuce Wraps

INGREDIENT

- 2 grilled chicken breasts, sliced
- 4 large lettuce leaves (such as romaine or butter lettuce)
- 1 ripe avocado, sliced
- 1/2 cup diced tomatoes
- 1/4 cup diced red onion
- Fresh cilantro leaves for garnish
- Lime wedges for serving

PREPARATION

- Place the grilled chicken slices in the center of each lettuce leaf.
- Top with sliced avocado, diced tomatoes, and diced red onion.
- Garnish with fresh cilantro leaves.
- Squeeze fresh lime juice over the filling.
- Roll up the lettuce leaves to form wraps.
- Serve the grilled chicken and avocado lettuce wraps as a light and flavorful lunch option.

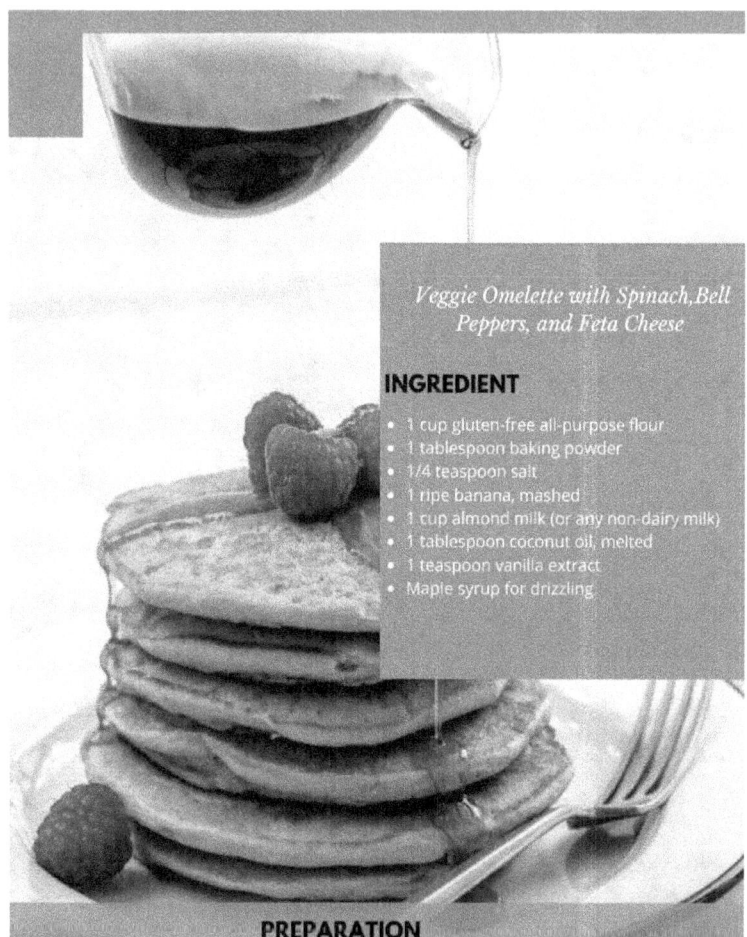

Veggie Omelette with Spinach, Bell Peppers, and Feta Cheese

INGREDIENT

- 1 cup gluten-free all-purpose flour
- 1 tablespoon baking powder
- 1/4 teaspoon salt
- 1 ripe banana, mashed
- 1 cup almond milk (or any non-dairy milk)
- 1 tablespoon coconut oil, melted
- 1 teaspoon vanilla extract
- Maple syrup for drizzling

PREPARATION

- In a mixing bowl, combine the gluten-free all-purpose flour, baking powder, and salt.
- In a separate bowl, mash the ripe banana until smooth.
- Add the mashed banana, almond milk, melted coconut oil, and vanilla extract to the dry ingredients. Stir until well combined.
- Heat a non-stick skillet or griddle over medium heat and lightly grease it with coconut oil or cooking spray.

- Pour about 1/4 cup of the pancake batter onto the skillet for each pancake.
- Cook until bubbles form on the surface of the pancakes, then flip them and cook for an additional 1-2 minutes, until golden brown.
- Repeat with the remaining batter.
- Serve the gluten-free banana pancakes with a drizzle of maple syrup.
- Enjoy the fluffy and delicious pancakes for a satisfying breakfast or brunch option.

INGREDIENT

- For the turkey meatballs:
- 1 pound ground turkey
- 1/4 cup almond flour (or breadcrumbs)
- 1/4 cup grated Parmesan cheese
- 1/4 cup chopped fresh parsley
- 1 clove garlic, minced
- 1/2 teaspoon dried oregano
- 1/2 teaspoon dried basil
- Salt and pepper to taste
- Olive oil for cooking
- For the homemade marinara sauce:
- 1 tablespoon olive oil
- 1 onion, chopped
- 2 cloves garlic, minced
- 1 can (400g) crushed tomatoes
- 1 teaspoon dried basil
- 1 teaspoon dried oregano
- Salt and pepper to taste
- 2-3 medium zucchini, spiralized or cut into noodles
- Fresh basil for garnish

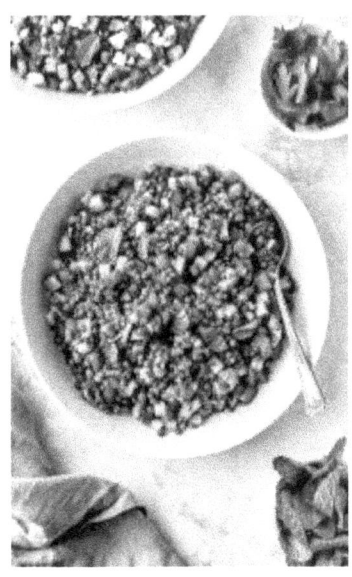

PREPARATION

- In a large bowl, combine the ground turkey, almond flour, grated Parmesan cheese, chopped fresh parsley, minced garlic, dried oregano, dried basil, salt, and pepper. Mix well until all the ingredients are evenly incorporated.
- Roll the turkey mixture into small meatballs, about 1 inch in diameter.
- Heat a little olive oil in a large skillet over medium heat.
- Add the turkey meatballs to the skillet and cook until they are browned on all sides and cooked through, about 10-12 minutes.
- While the meatballs are cooking, prepare the homemade marinara sauce. In a separate saucepan, heat the olive oil over medium heat.
- Add the chopped onion and minced garlic. Sauté until the onion is softened and translucent.
- Add the crushed tomatoes, dried basil, dried oregano, salt, and pepper to the saucepan. Stir well to combine.
- Reduce the heat to low and let the marinara sauce simmer for about 15-20 minutes, allowing the flavors to meld together.
- In a separate skillet, heat a little olive oil over medium heat.
- Add the zucchini noodles to the skillet and cook for about 2-3 minutes, until they are slightly softened but still retain some crunch.
- Remove the zucchini noodles from the heat.
- To serve, plate the zucchini noodles and top with turkey meatballs.
- Spoon the homemade marinara sauce over the meatballs and noodles.
- Garnish with fresh basil.
- Enjoy the flavorful and low-carb zucchini noodles with turkey meatballs and homemade marinara sauce for a satisfying dinner option.

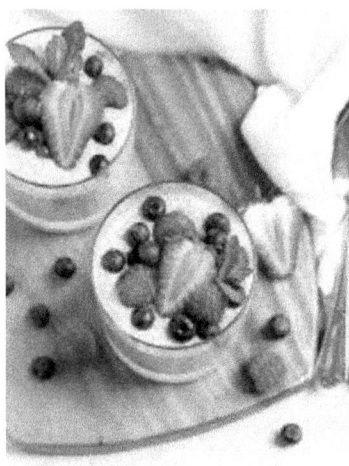

INGREDIENT

- 1 cup dried lentils (any variety)
- 4 cups vegetable broth
- 1 onion, chopped
- 2 carrots, diced
- 2 celery stalks, diced
- 2 cloves garlic, minced
- 1 teaspoon cumin
- 1 teaspoon paprika
- 1/2 teaspoon turmeric
- Salt and pepper to taste
- Fresh parsley for garnish
- For the mixed greens salad:
- Mixed salad greens
- Cherry tomatoes, halved
- Cucumber, sliced
- Red onion, thinly sliced

PREPARATION

- Rinse the lentils under cold water and drain.
- In a large pot, heat a little olive oil over medium heat.
- Add the chopped onion, diced carrots, and diced celery. Sauté until the vegetables are softened.
- Add the minced garlic, cumin, paprika, and turmeric. Stir well to coat the vegetables in the spices.
- Pour in the vegetable broth and add the rinsed lentils.
- Bring the mixture to a boil, then reduce the heat to low and simmer for about 25-30 minutes, or until the lentils are tender.
- Season the lentil soup with salt and pepper to taste.
- While the soup is simmering, prepare the mixed greens salad by combining the salad greens, cherry tomatoes, cucumber, and red onion in a bowl.
- Drizzle with balsamic vinaigrette dressing if desired.
- Serve the lentil soup with a side of mixed greens salad.
- Garnish the soup with fresh parsley.
- Enjoy the hearty and nutritious lentil soup with a refreshing mixed greens salad for a satisfying lunch or dinner.

Overnight Chia Pudding with Coconut Milk, topped with Fresh Berries and a sprinkle of Coconut Flakes

INGREDIENT

- 2 tablespoons chia seeds
- 1/2 cup coconut milk
- 1 tablespoon honey or maple syrup
- 1/2 teaspoon vanilla extract
- Fresh berries (such as strawberries, blueberries, and raspberries)
- Coconut flakes

PREPARATION

- In a jar or container, combine the chia seeds, coconut milk, honey or maple syrup, and vanilla extract.
- Stir well to ensure the chia seeds are evenly distributed.
- Cover the jar or container and refrigerate overnight or for at least 4 hours, allowing the chia seeds to absorb the liquid and thicken.
- In the morning, give the chia pudding a good stir.
- Serve the chia pudding in a bowl or glass, and top with fresh berries and a sprinkle of coconut flakes.
- Enjoy the creamy and nutritious overnight chia pudding for a satisfying breakfast.

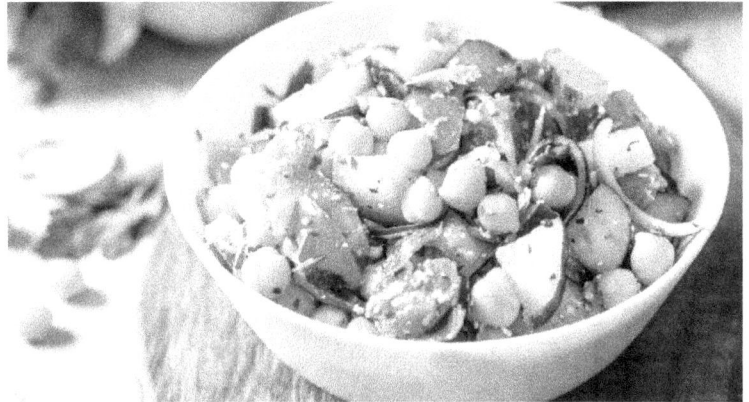

Chickpea Salad with Lemon-Tahini Dressing, served over a bed of Mixed Greens

INGREDIENT

- For the chickpea salad:
- 1 can (400g) chickpeas, rinsed and drained
- 1 cucumber, diced
- 1 red bell pepper, diced
- 1/4 red onion, finely chopped
- 1/4 cup chopped fresh parsley
- 1/4 cup chopped fresh mint
- For the lemon-tahini dressing:
- 2 tablespoons tahini
- 2 tablespoons lemon juice
- 1 tablespoon olive oil
- 1 clove garlic, minced
- Salt and pepper to taste
- Mixed salad greens

PREPARATION

- In a large bowl, combine the chickpeas, diced cucumber, diced red bell pepper, finely chopped red onion, chopped fresh parsley, and chopped fresh mint. Mix well.
- In a separate small bowl, whisk together the tahini, lemon juice, olive oil, minced garlic, salt, and pepper to make the lemon-tahini dressing.
- Pour the lemon-tahini dressing over the chickpea salad and toss until all the ingredients are coated.
- Place a bed of mixed salad greens on a plate or in a bowl.
- Spoon the chickpea salad over the mixed greens.
- Serve the refreshing and nutritious chickpea salad with lemon-tahini dressing as a light and satisfying lunch or dinner option.

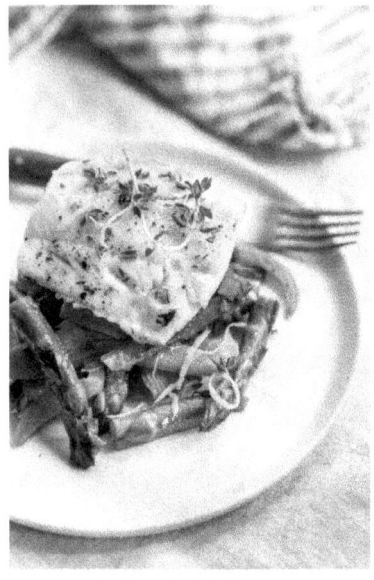

Baked Cod with Roasted Asparagus and Quinoa

INGREDIENT

- 2 cod fillets
- 1 tablespoon olive oil
- 1 lemon, sliced
- Salt and pepper to taste
- For the roasted asparagus:
- 1 bunch asparagus, trimmed
- 1 tablespoon olive oil
- Salt and pepper to taste
- Cooked quinoa for serving

PREPARATION

- Preheat the oven to 400°F (200°C).
- Place the cod fillets on a baking sheet lined with parchment paper.
- Drizzle the cod fillets with olive oil and squeeze fresh lemon juice over them.
- Season with salt and pepper to taste.
- Place lemon slices on top of the cod fillets.
- Bake the cod in the preheated oven for about 12-15 minutes, or until the fish is cooked through and flakes easily with a fork.
- While the cod is baking, prepare the roasted asparagus.
- Place the trimmed asparagus on a separate baking sheet.
- Drizzle with olive oil and season with salt and pepper.
- Toss the asparagus to coat it evenly with the oil and seasonings.
- Roast the asparagus in the oven for about 10-12 minutes, or until it is tender and slightly browned.
- Remove the cod and asparagus from the oven.
- Serve the baked cod with roasted asparagus and cooked quinoa.

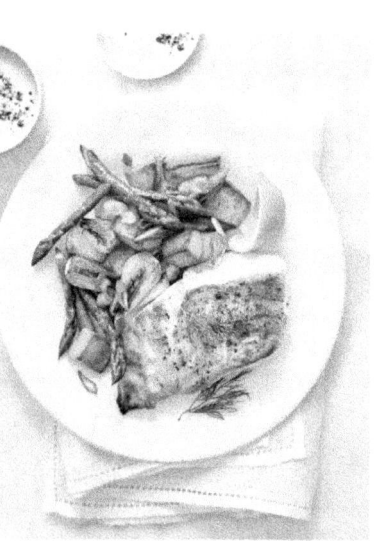

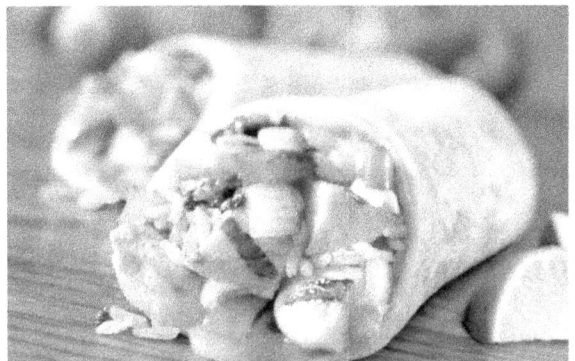

*Grilled Chicken and Avocado Wrap with
Lettuce, Tomato, and Greek Yogurt
Dressing*

INGREDIENT

- 2 grilled chicken breasts, sliced
- 2 whole wheat or gluten-free tortillas
- 1 avocado, sliced
- Lettuce leaves
- Tomato slices
- For the Greek yogurt dressing:
- 1/2 cup Greek yogurt
- 1 tablespoon lemon juice
- 1 tablespoon chopped fresh dill
- Salt and pepper to taste

PREPARATION

- In a small bowl, mix together the Greek yogurt, lemon juice, chopped fresh dill, salt, and pepper to make the Greek yogurt dressing.
- Lay out the tortillas and spread a generous amount of Greek yogurt dressing on each one.
- Top with sliced grilled chicken, avocado slices, lettuce leaves, and tomato slices.
- Roll up the tortillas tightly to form wraps.
- Slice the wraps in half, if desired.
- Serve the grilled chicken and avocado wraps as a satisfying and flavorful lunch or dinner option.

Green Smoothie Bowl with Spinach, Pineapple, and Almond Milk, topped with Fresh Berries and Granola

INGREDIENT

- 2 grilled chicken breasts, sliced
- 2 whole wheat or gluten-free tortillas
- 1 avocado, sliced
- Lettuce leaves
- Tomato slices
- For the Greek yogurt dressing:
- 1/2 cup Greek yogurt
- 1 tablespoon lemon juice
- 1 tablespoon chopped fresh dill
- Salt and pepper to taste

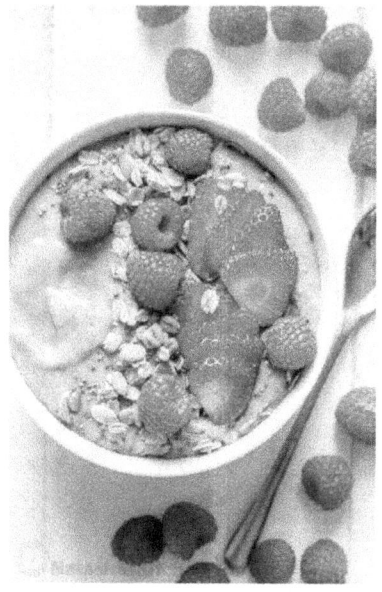

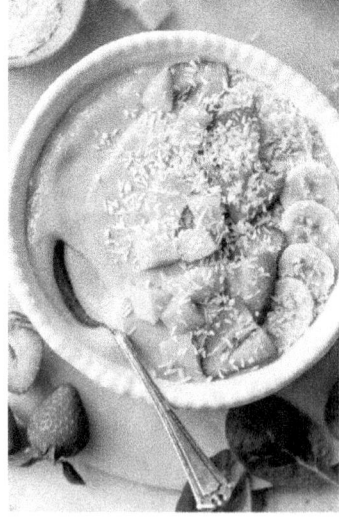

PREPARATION

- In a small bowl, mix together the Greek yogurt, lemon juice, chopped fresh dill, salt, and pepper to make the Greek yogurt dressing.
- Lay out the tortillas and spread a generous amount of Greek yogurt dressing on each one.
- Top with sliced grilled chicken, avocado slices, lettuce leaves, and tomato slices.
- Roll up the tortillas tightly to form wraps.
- Slice the wraps in half, if desired.
- Serve the grilled chicken and avocado wraps as a satisfying and flavorful lunch or dinner option.

Baked Salmon with Quinoa Pilaf and Steamed Broccoli

INGREDIENT

- 2 salmon fillets
- 1 tablespoon olive oil
- Salt and pepper to taste
- For the quinoa pilaf:
- 1 cup quinoa, rinsed
- 2 cups vegetable broth
- 1/4 cup chopped red onion
- 1/4 cup chopped bell pepper
- 1/4 cup chopped carrot
- 1/4 cup chopped zucchini
- 1/4 cup chopped mushrooms
- 1 clove garlic, minced
- 1 tablespoon olive oil
- Salt and pepper to taste
- Steamed broccoli florets for serving

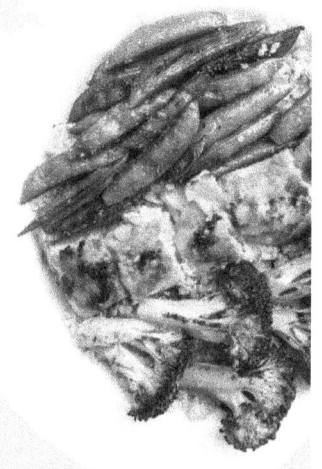

PREPARATION

- Preheat the oven to 400°F (200°C).
- Place the salmon fillets on a baking sheet lined with parchment paper.
- Drizzle the salmon fillets with olive oil and season with salt and pepper.
- Bake the salmon in the preheated oven for about 12-15 minutes, or until it is cooked through and flakes easily with a fork.
- While the salmon is baking, prepare the quinoa pilaf.
- In a saucepan, bring the vegetable broth to a boil. Add the rinsed quinoa and reduce the heat to low.
- Cover the saucepan and simmer for about 15-20 minutes, or until the quinoa is cooked and the liquid is absorbed.
- In a separate pan, heat the olive oil over medium heat. Add the chopped red onion, bell pepper, carrot, zucchini, mushrooms, and minced garlic.
- Sauté the vegetables until they are tender.
- Add the cooked quinoa to the pan with the sautéed vegetables. Season with salt and pepper

Rice Cakes with Almond Butter

INGREDIENT

- Rice cakes
- Almond butter

PREPARATION

- Take a rice cake and spread a generous amount of almond butter on top.
- Repeat with the remaining rice cakes.
- Serve the rice cakes with almond butter as a crunchy and nutritious snack option.

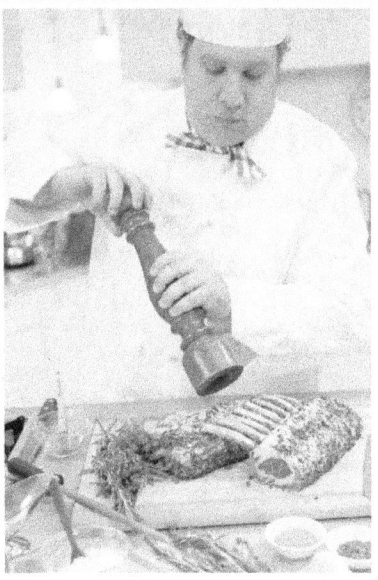

Mediterranean-Style Tuna Salad with Greek Yogurt Dressing

INGREDIENT

- 1 can tuna, drained
- 1/4 cup diced cucumber
- 1/4 cup diced tomato
- 1/4 cup diced red onion
- 1/4 cup diced Kalamata olives
- 1 tablespoon chopped fresh parsley
- For the Greek yogurt dressing:
- 1/4 cup Greek yogurt
- 1 tablespoon lemon juice
- 1 tablespoon chopped fresh dill
- Salt and pepper to taste

PREPARATION

- In a bowl, combine the drained tuna, diced cucumber, diced tomato, diced red onion, diced Kalamata olives, and chopped fresh parsley.
- In a separate small bowl, mix together the Greek yogurt, lemon juice, chopped fresh dill, salt, and pepper to make the Greek yogurt dressing.
- Pour the Greek yogurt dressing over the tuna salad mixture.
- Toss the salad until the ingredients are well coated with the dressing.
- Serve the Mediterranean-style tuna salad as a satisfying and protein-rich lunch or light dinner option.

Cottage Cheese with Sliced Peaches

INGREDIENT

- 1 cup cottage cheese
- 1 ripe peach, sliced

PREPARATION

- In a bowl, scoop the cottage cheese.
- Arrange the sliced peaches on top of the cottage cheese.
- Serve the cottage cheese with sliced peaches as a simple and protein-packed snack or light breakfast option.

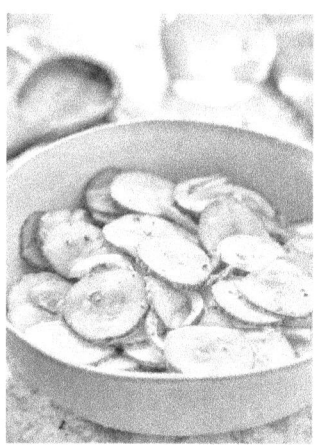
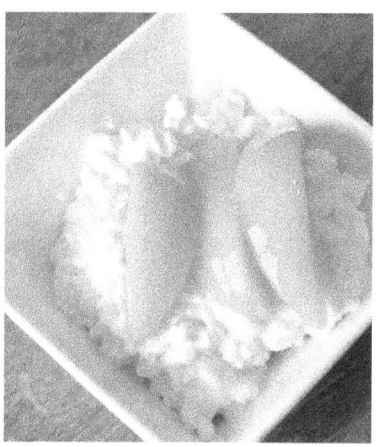

Cucumber Slices with Tzatziki Sauce

INGREDIENT

- 1 cucumber, sliced
- For the tzatziki sauce:
- 1 cup Greek yogurt
- 1/2 cucumber, grated
- 1 clove garlic, minced

PREPARATION

- In a small bowl, combine the Greek yogurt, grated cucumber, minced garlic, lemon juice, chopped fresh dill, salt, and pepper to make the tzatziki sauce.
- Arrange the cucumber slices on a plate or serving platter.
- Drizzle the tzatziki sauce over the cucumber slices.
- Serve the refreshing cucumber slices with tzatziki sauce as a light and healthy snack or appetizer.

Conclusion

"Cooking for PCOS Wellness: Nurturing Your Body with Satisfying and Nourishing Recipes" is more than just a cookbook. It is a powerful tool designed to empower individuals with Polycystic Ovary Syndrome (PCOS) to take control of their health, embrace their bodies, and thrive through the art of cooking and mindful eating. Throughout the chapters, we have explored a wide array of recipes, each carefully crafted to support PCOS management, nourish the body, and delight the taste buds.

By understanding the unique challenges of PCOS and the role of nutrition in managing its symptoms, this book offers a comprehensive approach to wellness. We have delved into the essential nutrients that support hormone balance and overall well-being, guiding you towards building a balanced PCOS-friendly diet.

From energizing breakfast delights and wholesome lunches to satisfying dinners, snacks, and sweet treats, this cookbook is filled with a diverse range of recipes that make healthy eating enjoyable and sustainable.

Beyond the recipes, this book has also explored the importance of mindfulness in eating habits and overcoming emotional eating challenges.

We have provided strategies for mindful meal planning, portion control, and building a healthy relationship with food and your body. The guidance on meal planning, shopping tips, and stocking your pantry with PCOS-friendly ingredients ensures that you have the tools and knowledge to make informed choices while navigating the grocery store and staying organized in your culinary journey.

Through this book, our aim has been to inspire and empower you to embrace cooking as a means of self-care and nourishment. We believe that by making conscious choices about what we put into our bodies, we can positively impact our PCOS symptoms, enhance our overall well-being, and cultivate a deep sense of self-love and acceptance.

Remember, this journey is unique to you. Each recipe, each ingredient, and each mindful bite is a step towards reclaiming your health and finding joy in the nourishment of your body. As you embark on this culinary adventure, we encourage you to listen to your body, honor its needs, and savor every moment spent in the kitchen.

May this book serve as a trusted companion, guiding you towards a harmonious relationship with food, promoting PCOS wellness, and igniting a lifelong love affair with delicious, satisfying, and nourishing meals? Embrace the power of cooking, savor the flavors, and let each meal be a celebration of your journey towards PCOS wellness and overall vitality.

Wishing you abundant health, happiness, and fulfillment on your path to PCOS wellness with love and nourishment

END!